FOOT REFLEXOLOGY

A Visual Guide for Self-Treatment

JÜRGEN JORA

ST. MARTIN'S PRESS
NEW YORK

FOOT REFLEXOLOGY. Copyright © 1991 by Tu-Ego-Verlag. All rights
reserved. Printed in Singapore. No part of this book may be used
or reproduced in any manner whatsoever without written permis-
sion except in the case of brief quotations embodied in critical ar-
ticles or reviews. For information, address St. Martin's Press, 175
Fifth Avenue, New York, N.Y. 10010.

Originally published in Germany under the title *Das Tu Ego Meth-
ode*, by Tu-Ego-Verlag, 1988.

Library of Congress Cataloging-in-Publication Data

Jora, Jürgen.
    [Tu-Ego-Methode-Buch. English]
    Foot reflexology: a visual guide for self-treatment /Jürgen Jora.
        p.   cm.
    Translation of: Das Tu-Ego-Methode-Buch.
    ISBN 0-312-05864-0 (pbk.)
    1. Reflexotherapy.   2. Foot—Massage.   I. Title.
    RM723.R43J6713   1991   90-28555
    615.8'22—dc20   CIP

First U.S. Edition: August 1991
10 9 8 7 6 5 4 3

Preface

Dear Readers,

I'm extremely pleased to present this book on the art of foot reflexology, a centuries-old art practiced by professional therapists and laypeople throughout the world.

The book is based on the numerous discoveries that I have made in more than ten years as a practicing foot reflexologist, and all of the examples described and illustrated herein are taken from my practice. The technique that I have developed (in Germany it is called the Tu-Ego, or "you-I" Method) is based on reflex-zone foot massage and sport massage. It is incredibly simple, and my successes to date in alleviating pain and eliminating the cause of disease have far exceeded my expectations. If you apply the suggested procedures correctly, and if you follow all of the book's recommendations, I believe that you will achieve much the same results, and that you will be surprised by the amazing natural power of your body to heal itself and to remain healthy and free of disease and pain.

A few words on the many supposedly incurable diseases: In my opinion there are none—they're just insufficiently understood! What's more, no one is infallible. Many wrong diagnoses are made. I'm certain nature has a cure for everything. It's only a matter of finding it and applying it correctly!

The Tu-Ego Method is based on reflex-zone foot massage. Show me a person whose feet are totally without calluses, without injuries, without hardenings, without knots, and I'll show you a completely healthy person!

I also expressly recommend my method to all nonmedical practitioners and naturopaths so that they, too, can be more successful in their occupations. Needless to say, I'd also be happy if open-minded general physicians adopted the Tu-Ego Method as well. I believe it would benefit all patients.

Wishing you the best of success with the Tu-Ego Method,

Yours truly,

Jürgen Jora

Introduction

The foot reflexology method described in this book is a further development of reflex-zone foot massage using some sport massage and taking all the reflex zones of the human body into account.

In general: If at all possible, the method should be practiced by two people—an active and a passive partner. Self-treatment should be practiced only when absolutely necessary, since only a passive partner can really relax.

Important: Alcohol should be avoided during the entire treatment phase, thus multiplying the effectiveness of the method. Alcohol paralyzes the central nervous system and definitely hinders the healing process. Unless your doctor advises otherwise, you should eat normally. Dieting or fasting is inappropriate because the body requires well-balanced, nutritional meals during the treatment period.

The History of Reflex-Zone Foot Massage

It's sad but true: Our feet, on which our whole body rests, are largely neglected even though they affect our entire well-being. Just as roots are important to a plant, feet are important to human beings. They're a wonder of nature but receive little attention.

Like so much else, foot massage originated in Asia. More than a thousand years ago, reflex-zone massage was recognized as a natural method of healing. It quickly fell into obscurity, however.

Or was it perhaps deliberately forgotten? Whatever the case, reflex-zone foot massage—via interested naturopaths and therapists using natural remedies—eventually made its way to Europe and America. It has been gratefully adopted in many countries, becoming a blessing for many people.

Unfortunately, a lot of physicians scoff at the practice of foot reflexology, relegate it to the realm of the mystical, and refuse to recognize it. But reflex-zone foot massage is the most powerful anti-disease weapon there is, and it's a *natural* weapon besides. I'd like to emphasize that it's not meant to replace doctors, but to spare them from having to deal with ailments not requiring their specialized knowledge.

This book will become a faithful companion, helping you to live a healthy, pain-free life.

A Word About Feet

Shoes were unknown to our ancient forefathers; they went barefoot. But we squeeze our feet into shoes, losing direct contact with the ground. It's a central problem. It may sound trivial, but by wearing shoes we deprive our organs of the benefits provided by the reflex zones on our feet. What's even worse, the lack of ventilation, and the constant pressure (caused by "fashionable" footwear that is often much too small) brings on calluses, corns, hammertoes, and other deformities.

Our society is probably more health conscious today than it ever was, so the importance of wearing the right shoes beginning in childhood shouldn't be news to anyone. Believe me, *if you try to cut corners when you buy shoes, you're cutting the wrong corners!*

But beware of so-called orthopedic shoes. Some are actually injurious to your health and aren't worthy of the name at all.

Your shoes should allow your body weight to be distributed over the entire foot. With some shoes, however, the weight is concentrated mainly on the joints of the toes, and this causes pinching, calluses, bunions, and often deformities on the sides of the big toes. A lifetime of wearing ill-fitting shoes can lead to arthritis, stiff feet, and a total loss of blood circulation to the foot area.

Even more problematic is the fact that these ailments may not stay confined to the feet, but can affect the entire body. It's a known fact that **the feet are a mirror image of the body** and contain, neurologically speaking, the same elements that make up the body as a whole. Each foot corresponds to exactly half of the body—right side to right foot, and left side to left foot. The exception is the head (eyes, sinuses, ears, etc.), whose reflex zones center in the big toes and sometimes the adjacent toes. In the case of the head, the nerve pathways seem to be transposed, that is, the right side of the head corresponds to the left foot; the left side to the right foot. The reflex zones of the teeth, however, are not transposed, i.e., left-side teeth correspond to left big toe, etc. The secret is simply to soften all of the hardness and knots in one's feet and to put them in good working order again by massaging the foot muscles. **If you return your feet to their original form, you'll eliminate the ailments.** So it becomes abundantly clear just how important it is that your feet can move naturally. Comfortable, flexible shoes are a must.

Tips: The above-mentioned ailments can be treated by massaging the feet once daily. In general, the feet should be massaged three times a week (or even better, every other day) until the reflex zones are completely free of pain.

I'd like to point out that reflex-zone foot massage isn't a therapeutic treatment, but simply an artificial way of going barefoot—a systematic way of going barefoot, of course. So anyone can do it—privately, that is. If it's done commercially, a license is required. **Only trained persons are permitted to practice massage professionally.**

Are There Hypochondriacs?

How often have you heard the phrase, "There's nothing medically wrong with him"? People who feel unwell, but who exhibit no observable, testable sign of illness have a rough time of it. Nobody believes them; their ailments are thought to be either feigned or imagined.

There are many such cases, and it has been my professional experience that these people are often extremely tense, up to their neck in work, or simply lonely. In some instances, however (this can be documented), such patients were completely pain-free after a single foot-massage session.

During reflex-zone foot massage, the reflex zones hurt immediately, unmistakable proof that the body has suffered some form of injury or illness or trauma. Put simply, your body never lies! And so there can be only one answer: There is no such thing as a hypochondriac!

A Healthy Person

A person's chances of avoiding disease are greater than many think. A lot of attention is paid nowadays to keeping clean and even aseptic, which is praiseworthy and important.

But an aseptic environment causes our body's defense mechanisms to grow inactive and weak. Children who grow up freely in a natural environment and are allowed to get dirty on occasion are much better equipped for later life than those who have been overprotected and shielded from everything.

We know that children who have gone through their so-called "childhood diseases" never come down with those illnesses again. Their bodies have formed the antibodies that immunize them for the rest of their lives.

Some people never even catch cold. They're said to be "tough," but are, in fact, among the lucky few whose bodily defenses are strong and who never get sick in their lives.

So there really are "perpetually healthy" people. You can strive to be one of them, too, by mobilizing your body's defense mechanisms. The most important step is to make sure that your organs function well and your muscles and joints are well supplied with blood. Massage focusing primarily on the feet activates all of the organs, leads to better blood circulation, helps balance the distribution of nutrients, promotes the disposal of waste products, and leads to a healthy, ailment-free body.

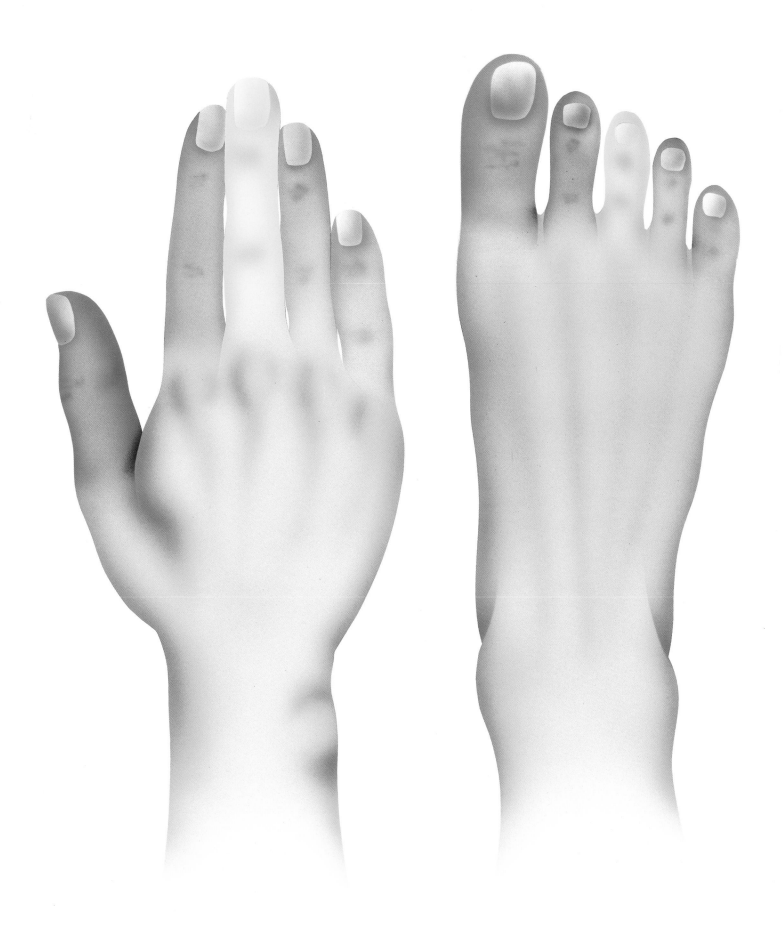

Foot Reflexology for the Hands and Feet

As the illustration at the left clearly shows, it is easy to find the various reflex zones (pain centers). Different colors have been used to indicate the correspondence between toes and fingers. The big toe corresponds to the thumb, the middle toe to the middle finger, et cetera.

If you have pain in your big toe, then massage your thumb and vice versa. If the injury has just occurred, the pain should subside or go away very quickly.

An example from the world of sports: A soccer player jams his big toe, spraining the joint. The masseur should immediately massage the thumb and knuckle. After about five minutes, the pain in the toe should subside, provided a bone isn't broken or a muscle torn, et cetera. The thumb and knuckle should be massaged intensively for about twenty minutes. In most cases, the athlete will then be ready to play again. The massage must be repeated daily until the toe is no longer discolored or until it can be moved without pain. In urgent cases, the area can be massaged twice daily. For the second massage, ten minutes is sufficient. This procedure is applicable to all injuries.

Here is another example of how the hand corresponds to the foot: A waiter with aching feet finds relief by rubbing his hands, vigorously kneading them until the pain in his feet is lessened and he can return to his customers.

How is it done? If the balls of your feet hurt, massage the corresponding part of your hands—the top part of the palm just below the fingers. If your ankles are sore, massage your wrists, etc. In short, whenever your foot aches, massage the corresponding part of your hand and vice versa. Duration of the massage: from five to twenty minutes.

Note: Anyone can find relief through massage. It's just a matter of practice.

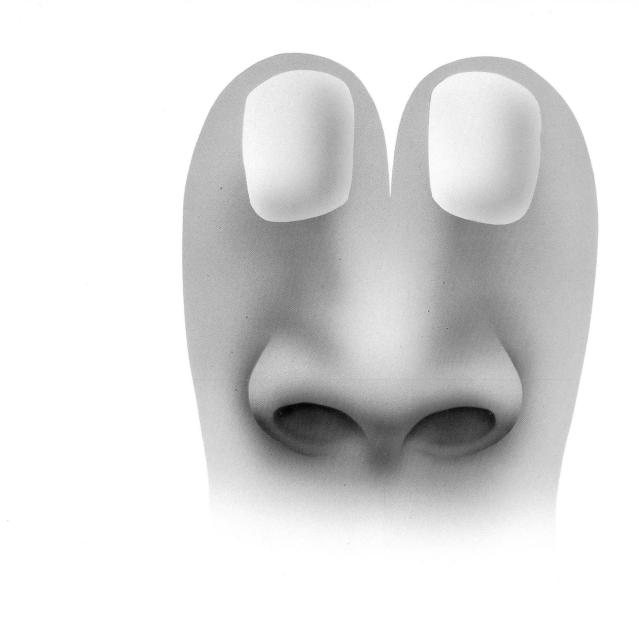

Foot Reflexology for the Nose and Nasal Sinuses

The unusual illustration of the nose at the top of the opposite page is meant to serve as a learning aid. You've probably already noticed that **the big toes are reversed,** indicating that the body's nervous system is "wired" crosswise! The lower illustration clearly shows that the right big toe corresponds to the sinuses on the left side of the face, and that the left big toe corresponds to the sinuses on the right side of the face. Treating the top, "upper," side of the big toes helps clear the nose and nasal sinuses.

Massage: Massage softly at first, slowly increasing the pressure. Later, you should use your thumbs to press down at various points on the toe.

Reactions: The person being treated may feel pain because this part of the toe is extremely sensitive. But it's better to feel some pain for a few minutes than to have to put up with a stuffed-up nose or congested nasal sinuses all day.

Duration of massage: About three minutes per toe. If performed properly, the massage will begin to show results even before it's completed.

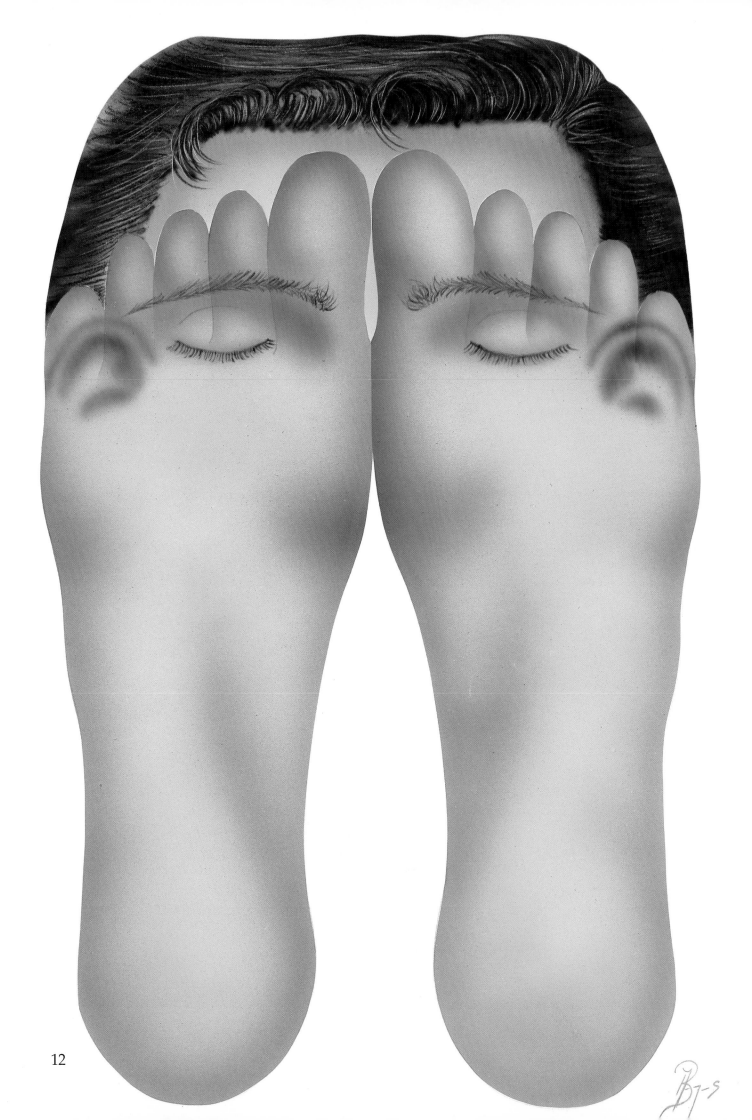

12

Foot Reflexology for the Upper Sinuses

The balls of your toes correspond to the upper sinuses. As stated above, the nerves are arranged crosswise. But you needn't pay attention to that as long as you always remember to massage both feet.

The best way to massage the balls of your toes is by squeezing them between your thumb and index finger (see illustration). When you have sinus trouble, it's also a good idea to massage the reflex zones of the nose and nasal sinuses as well (see page 10).

Note: If you feel pain on one side of your frontal sinuses, you should always massage the balls of your toes and cups of your fingers on the opposite foot or hand more intensively.

Rule: Always massage your hands and feet completely if possible, concentrating on the problem areas.

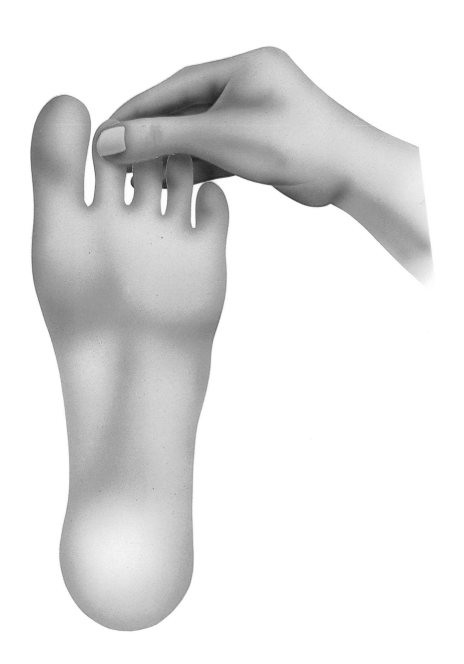

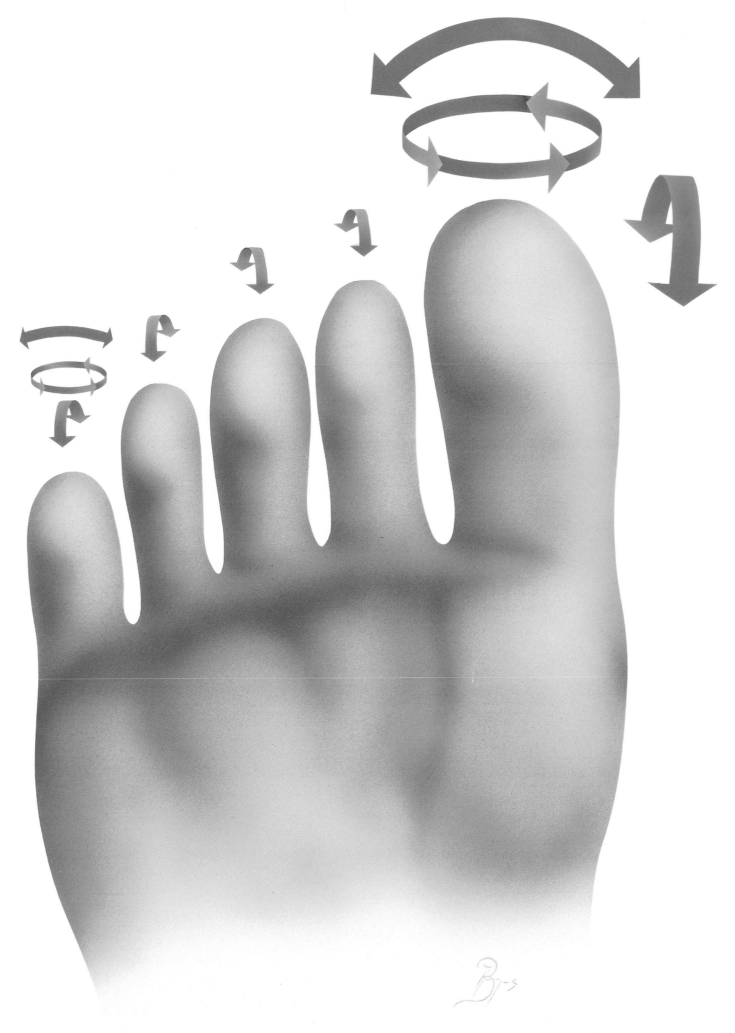

Foot Reflexology to Limber the Body

Whenever you have discomfort in your head, neck, shoulder, arm, or chest, the lower cervical vertebrae are involved. In other words, the vertebrae are jammed and must be limbered.

Limbering the cervical vertebrae can be accomplished by massaging the basal joint of the big toe. To do this, take the big toe of the right foot as shown below and move it back and forth. This should be continued until the patient feels resistance manifesting itself as pain. At that point, pressure must be released immediately (the patient should raise his hand to indicate when he feels pain).

The limbering procedure should initially be repeated three to four times. After that, you should try—as shown in the illustration at left—to describe circular movements. These should also be stopped as soon as they begin to cause pain.

In some cases, the toe will become limber immediately and allow itself to be moved freely. In many cases, however, it will grate and begin to hurt. If it does, stop momentarily, then try again, moving it from right to left and left to right. Repeat this three to four times, then apply the same procedure to the other foot.

Needless to say, these movements should always be performed very carefully but with a certain amount of pressure. Every person has a different threshold of pain. The two massage partners simply have to harmonize. Experienced therapists are familiar with these reactions, of course.

You can often recognize a jammed cervical vertebra by swelling of the basal joint (articular capsule) of the big toe and the presence of bunions.

After limbering—or trying to limber—the big toes, the other toes should be manipulated in the same way (note arrows).

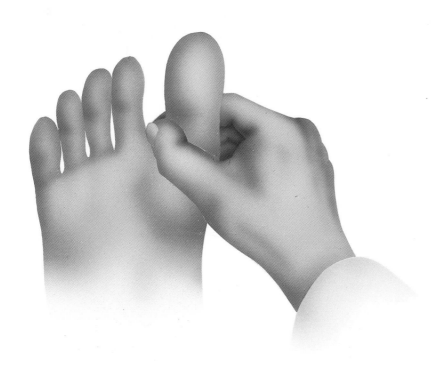

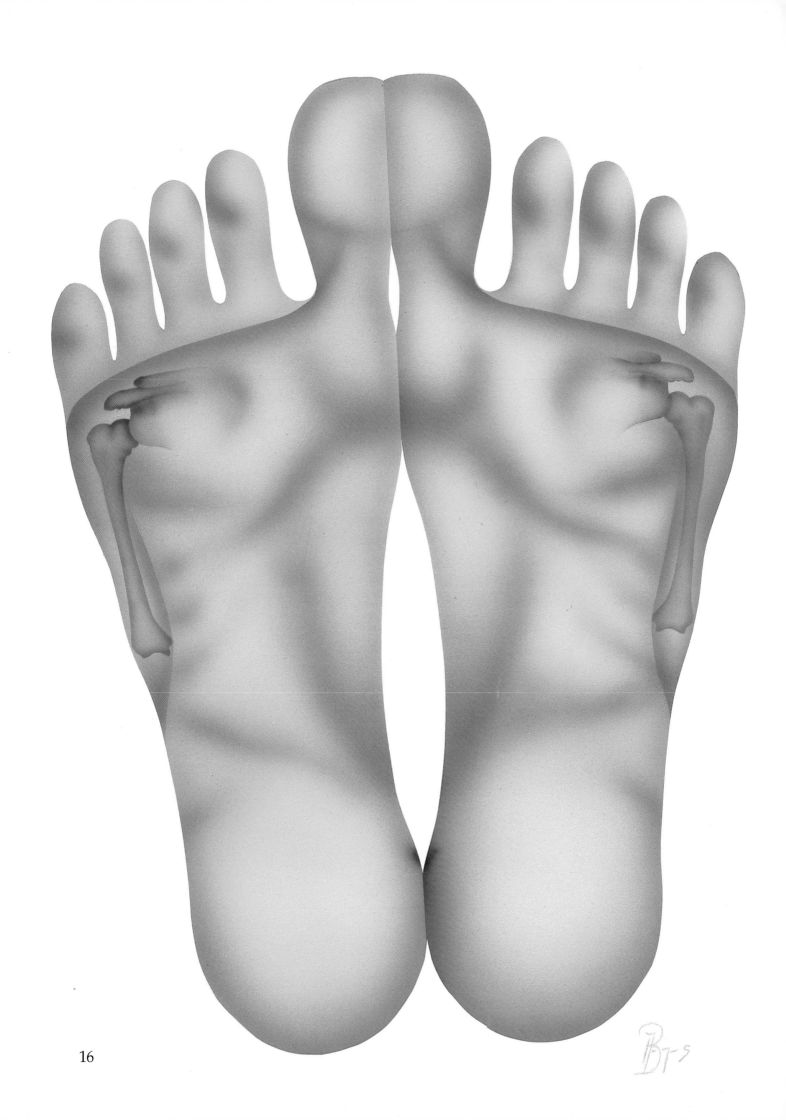

16

Foot Reflexology for the Shoulder Joint

By limbering the basal joint of the little toe, you affect the shoulder joint on the opposite side of the body (please note the illustration).

Important: Never use force in trying to move the toes. Always move them carefully until you meet resistance, and then press lightly. Don't forget to use the hand signal at the first sign of pain.

Experience has shown that massage every other day is sufficient. Any knot can be eliminated with time; just be patient!

Additional bodily reactions: When the basal joints of the big toes loosen, that is, allow themselves to be turned or bent to the left or right, your body will experience a rush of warmth, particularly in your head. This is an indication of improved circulation. General improvement will soon follow.

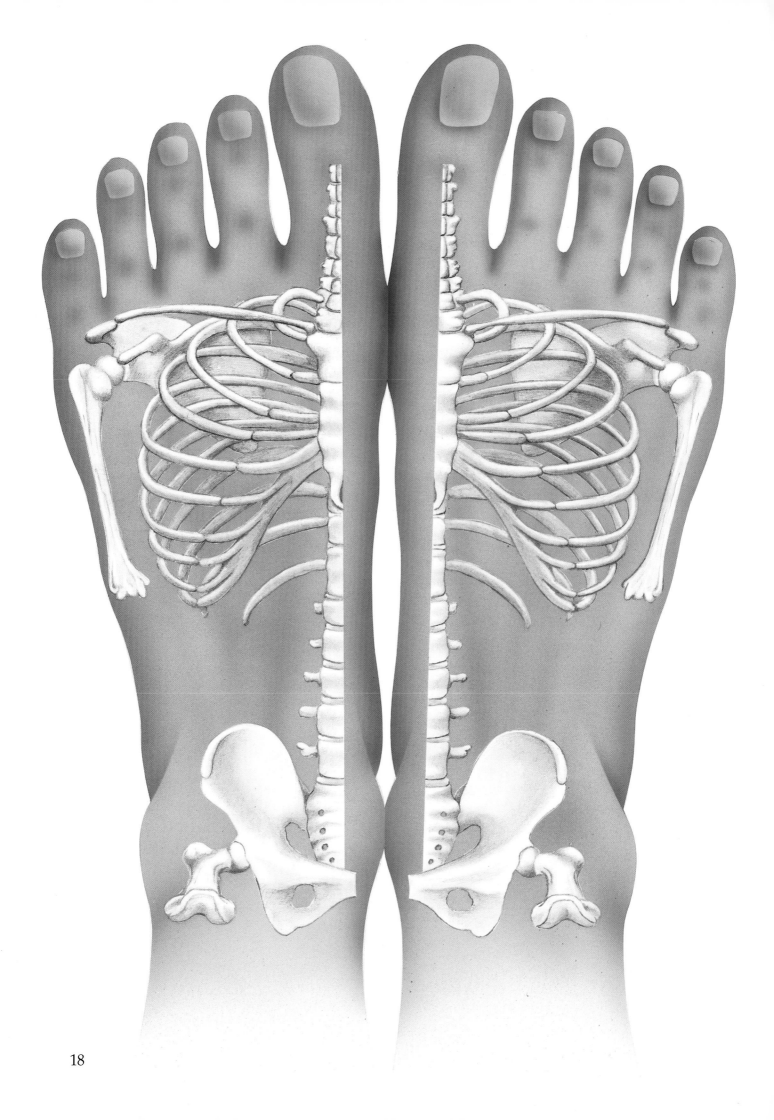

Foot Reflexology for the Spinal Column and Frontal Skeleton

The basal joint of the big toe is one of the most important reflex zones of all. A person whose basal joint is stiff or the site of a large bunion often suffers extreme discomfort, such as migraine headaches, dizziness, impaired circulation, sore neck or shoulder, numbness in the arms and hands.

If the basal joint of the big toe is stiff, badly swollen, or the site of a large bunion, the lower cervical vertebra is very strongly affected. These conditions can also indicate that other joints are undersupplied with blood, which can result in deposits and desiccation.

If circulation is chronically impaired, the head, shoulder, arms, and hands will be supplied with less and less blood and cleansed more infrequently of waste products.

Disorders of the neck, nose, eyes, and ears can result as well. Moreover, the direct reflex zone from the lower cervical vertebra to the lower lumbar vertebra becomes blocked, causing disorders of the lower extremities, too.

In short, the person becomes ill.

You can clearly see where to massage in the illustration on the opposite page. As you work on the foot, feel for swelling and hardness and massage lightly at first, increasing the pressure in accordance with the patient's threshold of pain. The massage should be repeated daily until all swelling, hardness, and knots have disappeared from the feet, indicating that the injury is most likely healed.

Note that the ankle is the reflex zone for the hip, knee, elbow, and wrist.

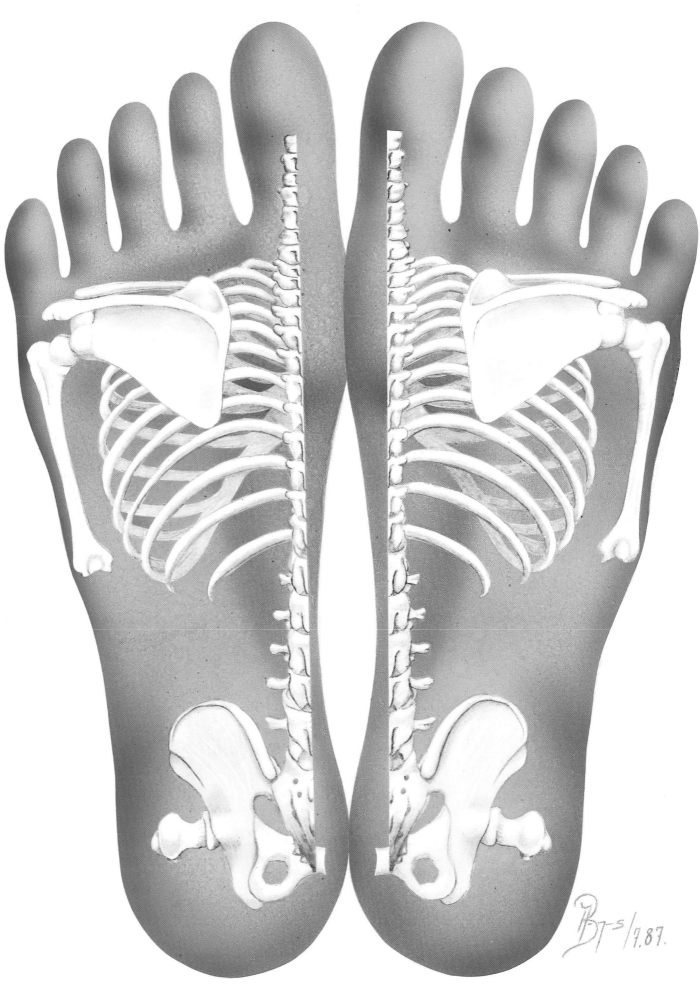

20

Foot Reflexology for the Spinal Column and Skeleton of the Back

The shoulders, which correspond to the basal joints of the little toes, are often the site of problems. You may feel knots here, and the skin is often calloused in these areas. If you apply pressure, you'll feel a stabbing pain—a sign that circulation is impaired.

You should massage your feet well every other day until all the knots have disappeared. A good technique is to apply pressure massage with the thumb. Sore shoulder muscles are a good indication of proper circulation.

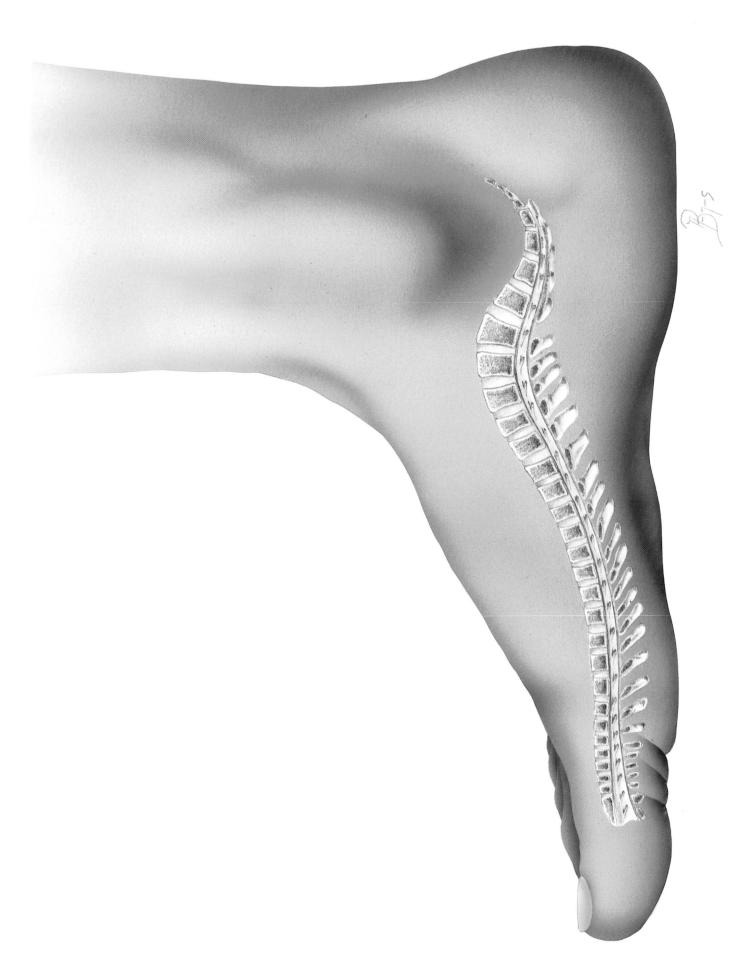

Foot Reflexology for the Spinal Column (a Cross-Section View)

The illustration at the left shows a cross-section of the spinal column and spinal cord. Optimal blood circulation in the spinal column is achieved by applying soft and sensitive massage to these zones. The first massage very often relieves the pain, especially in cases of recent injuries, dislocations, cramps, sciatica, incipient Bechterew's disease, and all acute discomfort regardless of its nature. It is advisable to massage the foot reflex zones for the spinal column whatever the problem. As you massage, remember to press gently rather than rub. Afterward, gently smooth out the area, always stroking toward the ankle.

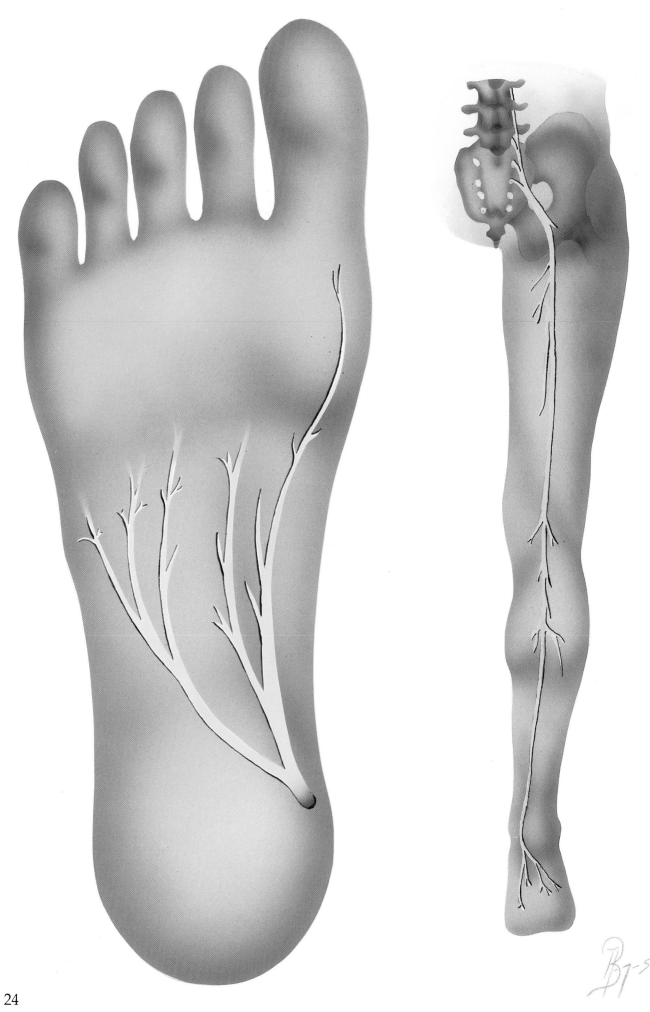

24

Foot Reflexology for Sciatica

This intensely painful condition can best be cured by vigorously massaging the zones marked in the illustration shown at left. They should be massaged until you have a pleasant sensation of warmth in your buttocks and back. This warmth can and may also be felt in your head.

Important: Massage both feet. The massage is quite painful but very effective.

The lumbar (lower back), sacrum, and coccyx (base of spine) regions should be massaged on both feet as well.

Note: Remember that the best massage always includes both feet. Massage *all* of both feet, paying particular attention to the problem zones. Don't forget the basal joints of the big toes! Also note the chapter on first aid and self-help.

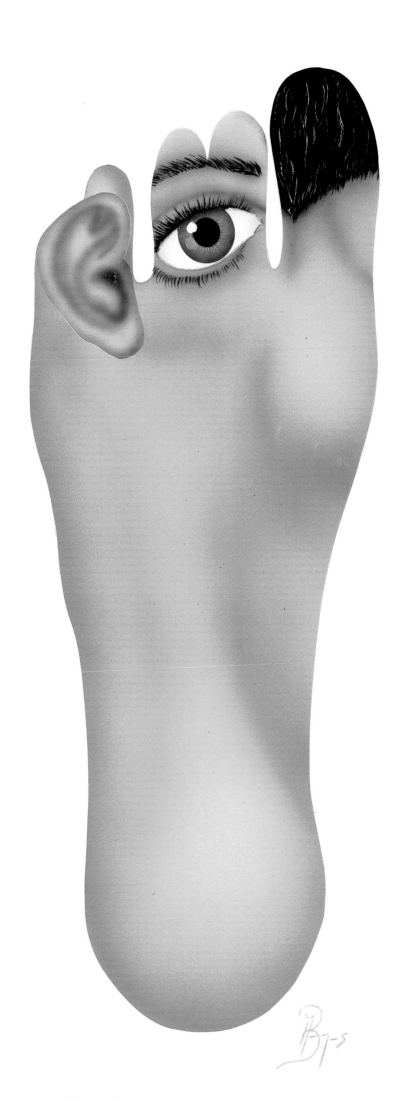

26

Foot Reflexology for the Eyes and Ears

Eye disorders: If the index and middle fingers or the second and third toes (reflex zones for the eyes) are misshapen, hardened, have little knots, or are injured, eye pain and disease can result.

Conversely, whatever affects the eyes is passed on to the reflex zones on the hands and feet. That means the reflex zones for the eyes will begin to swell, and the longer the eye disorder lasts, the harder the zones become.

If the eye is treated directly, but blood circulation in the reflex zones on the toes and fingers is inadequate, the knots will remain. Consequently, the eye disorder will most likely remain, too.

It is important to include the reflex zones for the eyes each time you massage the feet and hands. This creates a balance between blood supply and waste disposal in the eye, and may result in relief of eye pain and in improved vision. For all massages, it's important to limber the basal joints of the big toes first (lower cervical vertebra).

Don't get discouraged. Success has been achieved even in virtually hopeless cases. An improvement in vision, no matter how slight, is well worth the effort of a long-term program of hand and foot massage.

Ear disorders: Ear disorders are treated using the same procedure that applies to the eyes. Begin by loosening the basal joints of the big toes, then concentrate on the fourth toe and little toe. Your balance will probably improve, and you may notice a discharge from your ears (temporary self-cleaning). For more serious ear or eye disorders, you should contact your doctor.

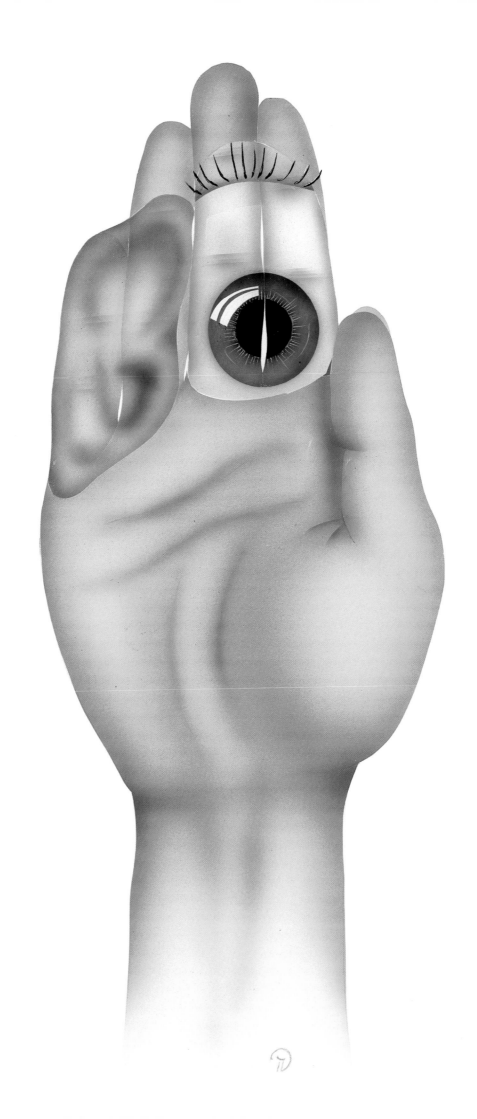

Hand Reflexology for the Eyes and Ears

Note: Always consult your doctor when you've injured an eye or an ear.

Massage: Note that the left eye and left ear correspond to the right hand and vice versa. Feel for the most sensitive spots in the reflex zones on the fingers and massage them without causing excessive pain. After a few moments, you may notice that the eye or ear pain has subsided somewhat. As a precautionary measure, keep massaging for a minute or two, repeating the procedure if necessary.

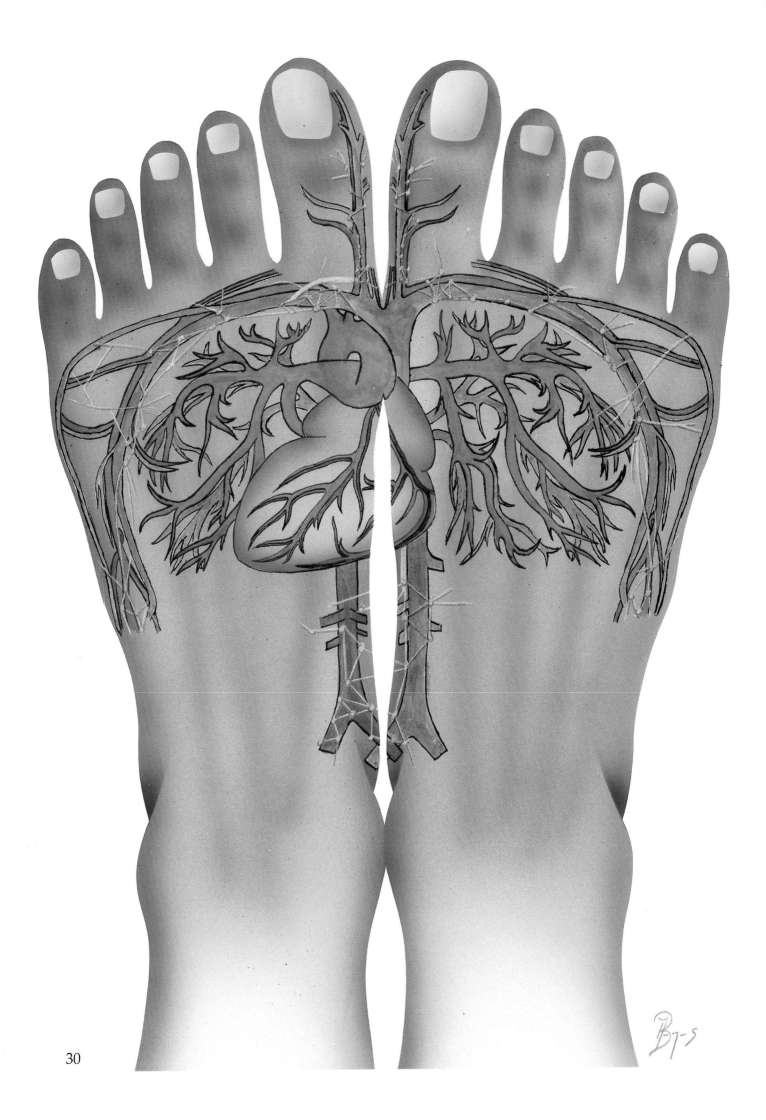

Foot Reflexology for the Heart and Circulatory System, the Lymph Vessels and Nodes

Your heart and circulatory system, as well as your lymph vessels and nodes, react wonderfully to reflex-zone massage. Massaging these areas is incredibly simple, and the results can be astounding.

By studying the illustration at left, it will become clear just how important the basal joints of the big toes are as a reflex zone. Limber this zone first, using the instructions on page 15. Then proceed to massage all of both feet, paying special attention to the reflex zones for the kidneys, urinary duct, bladder, and adrenal glands, all of which play a very important role in strengthening the heart. (See pages 40–41 for locating these zones.)

During the first week, it's advisable to massage daily, or at least every other day until there is no longer any swelling or hardness. Afterward, you should massage once a week as a preventative measure.

You should plan on about five minutes for each foot, although the session can be extended to fifteen minutes. When you start treatment, make sure that you don't overdo it. Massage softly at first and increase the pressure later.

Important: Remain sitting—or even better, lying—for at least five minutes after the massage. You might even take a short nap, which would be ideal.

Foot reflexology is not a substitute for professional medical care. See your doctor for regular checkups and if you have or think you may have a heart, circulatory, or lymphatic condition.

Note: When you wear shoes that are too tight or too high (particularly women's shoes), deposits quickly gather in the basal joints of the toes and may lead to disorders in the zones shown in the illustration.

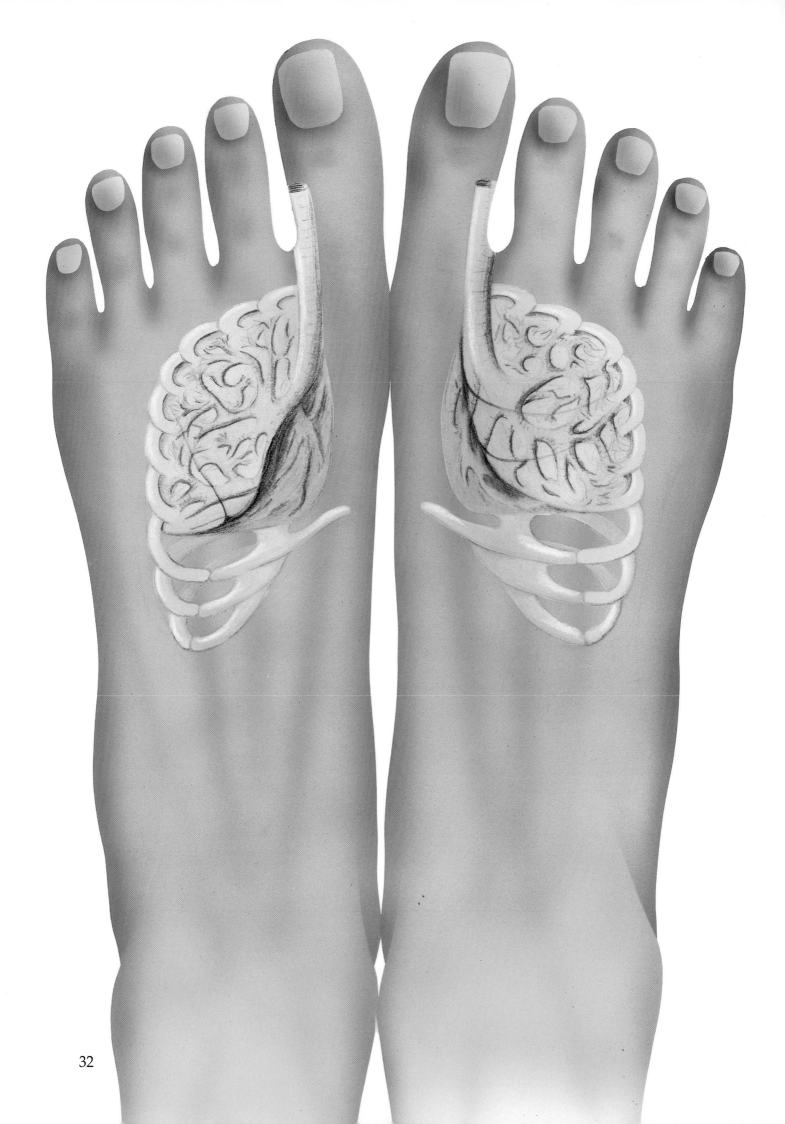

Foot Reflexology for the Lungs and Bronchial Tubes

We all know that problems with the bronchi—resulting in shortness of breath, constant wheezing, and pain—are extremely unpleasant. They can even bring on anxiety attacks. Coughing up accumulated phlegm brings no relief. Solving bronchial problems requires a lot of staying power, trust, and patience. It would help if you got rid of any emotional stress you might be feeling. Quarrels, tension, and irritation should be avoided (which is, of course, easier said than done).

The illustration at the left and the hand reflex-zone illustration on page 34 show where you massage for relief of bronchial problems. If possible, try to have someone else perform the massage.

Important: Always massage the area surrounding the designated zones, too. You should always start with the right foot; make sure to turn the illustrations to match the way your massage partner's feet are pointing at you!

In my practice I've often seen people who reacted negatively or whose bronchial condition even seemed to worsen. If this happens to you, try not to be alarmed. Your symptoms will most likely disappear over time, with regular application of reflex-zone massage. Trust and patience are important. That's surely not always easy, but your personal efforts should pay off. The constant massages will breathe new life into your body.

For all serious bronchial ailments, always consult your doctor.

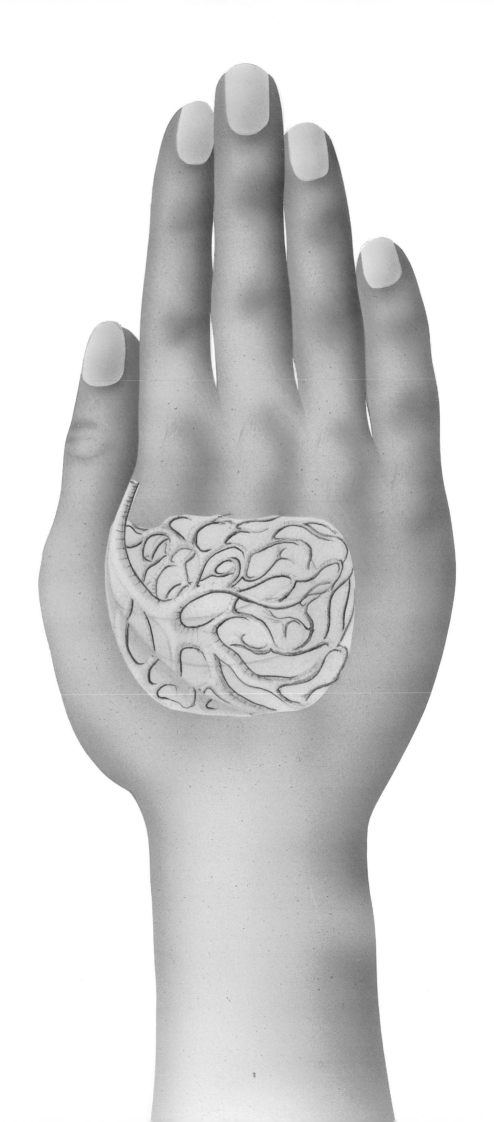

34

First Aid for Bronchial Discomfort

Whenever you're plagued by shortness of breath, coughing, and bronchial discomfort, immediately use your thumb to "pump" the area between the thumb and index finger shown in the illustration. Make sure to massage both hands. Afterward, massage the entire hands, using a circular motion, until you feel relief.

Remember, the reflex zones of the hand correspond to those of the foot.

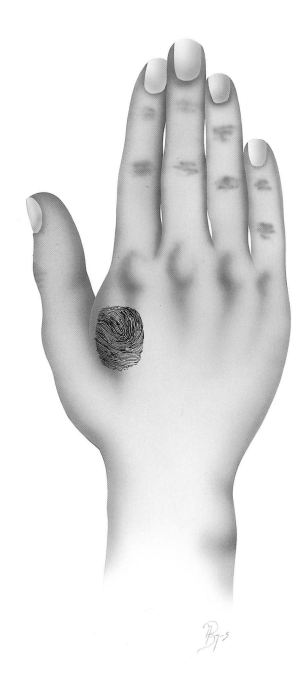

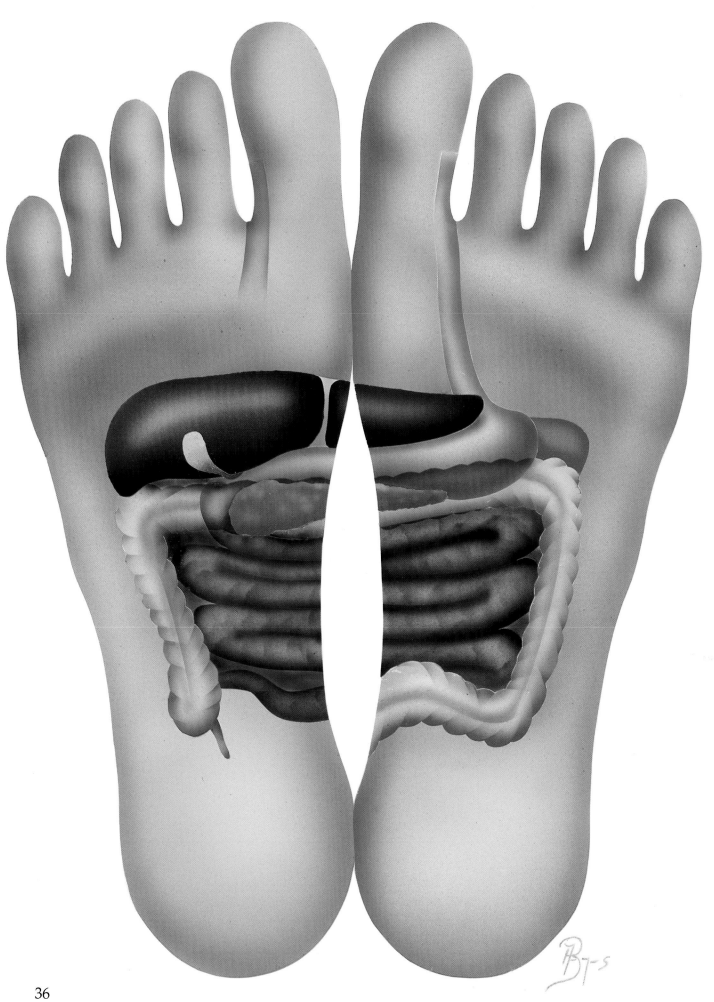

Foot Reflexology for the Liver, Gall Bladder, Esophagus, Stomach, Intestines, Pancreas, and Spleen

The illustration at left clearly shows how intertwined these organs are—all of them have similar functions. You can see the esophagus (twice: one on each foot), the stomach in the curve of the duodenum, and the pancreas (ending in the left foot). Under that is the small intestine and ileum (which opens into the large intestine), the appendix and vermiform appendix, the ascending colon, transverse colon, and descending colon.

Massage technique: Go softly and carefully at first, applying light pressure with the thumb. Massage the whole area, paying particular attention to the problem zones. Later, when the zones are not as sensitive (after several massages), apply more pressure, always being on the lookout for your partner's hand signals. Massage all organs softly. Never overdo it!

Consult your doctor for serious or persistent problems.

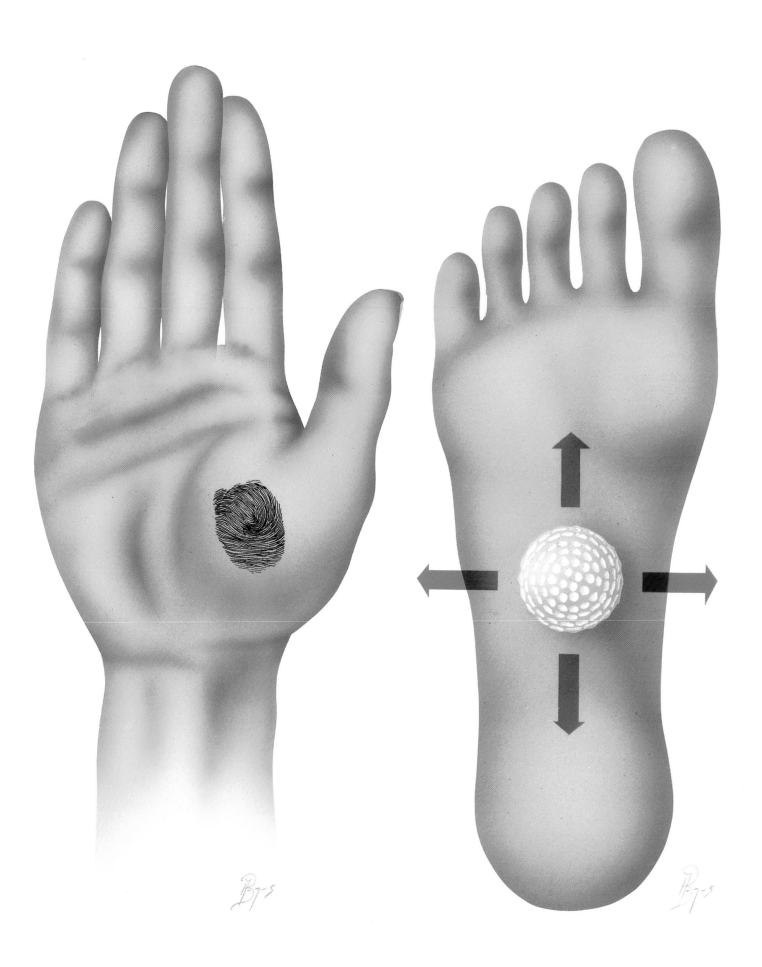

First Aid for Stomach Problems

Foot reflex-zone technique: For emergency relief of stomach discomfort, you can either stand on a golf ball or roll your foot over it, back and forth, left or right, and between your feet. If you're on the go (or don't have a golf ball), you can use the roundest and smoothest stone or other round object you can find. The illustration on page 51 shows another possibility for treatment. A piece of a broom handle or something similar will do. You're sure to find something.

Hand reflex-zone technique: When you have a stomachache, repeatedly press the balls of your hands below the basal joint of the thumb (the area of the fingerprint in the illustration at far left). You'll have to feel for the spot—it's rather far down. It will be the point that hurts the most. Pump this point (press, release, press, release) with your thumb for about two minutes. Your stomach should begin to warm and you'll probably begin to feel better. If necessary (should the pain continue), repeat the procedure.

Finally, I'd also like to recommend the use of a gravel-filled box, which is a great way to massage your feet. At first you can massage them in a sitting position. Later, when your feet have grown accustomed to the procedure, you can walk around in the box. But here again, don't overdo it.

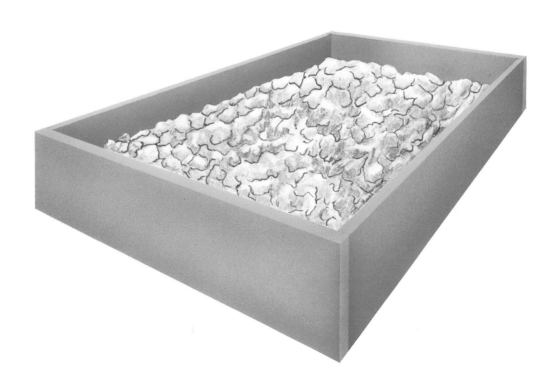

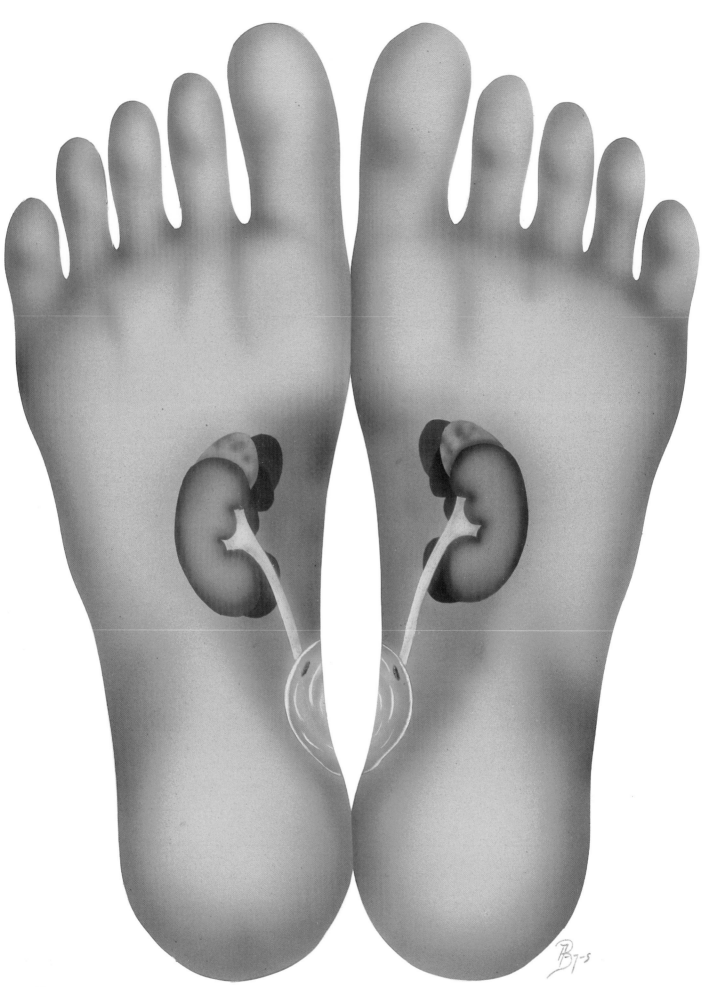

40

Foot Reflexology for the Kidneys, Adrenal Glands, Ureter, and Bladder

The reflex zones for the kidneys, adrenal glands, ureter, and bladder are adjacent to those of the spinal column (see illustration on page 22). It has been my experience that disorders of the spinal column almost always involve the adjacent organs. For example, if you have a kidney problem that hasn't been remedied, you're likely to have a spinal column disorder (and vice versa). If the spinal column is injured in an accident, the adjacent organ is often afflicted, too.

A consistent program of massage on the reflex points of the organs in question can help avert worse damage.

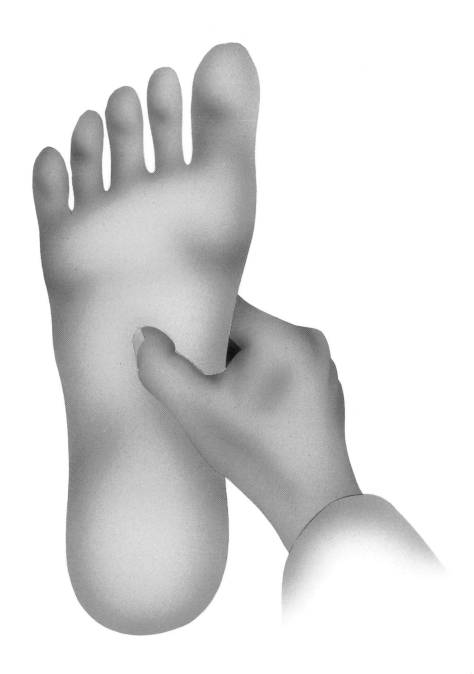

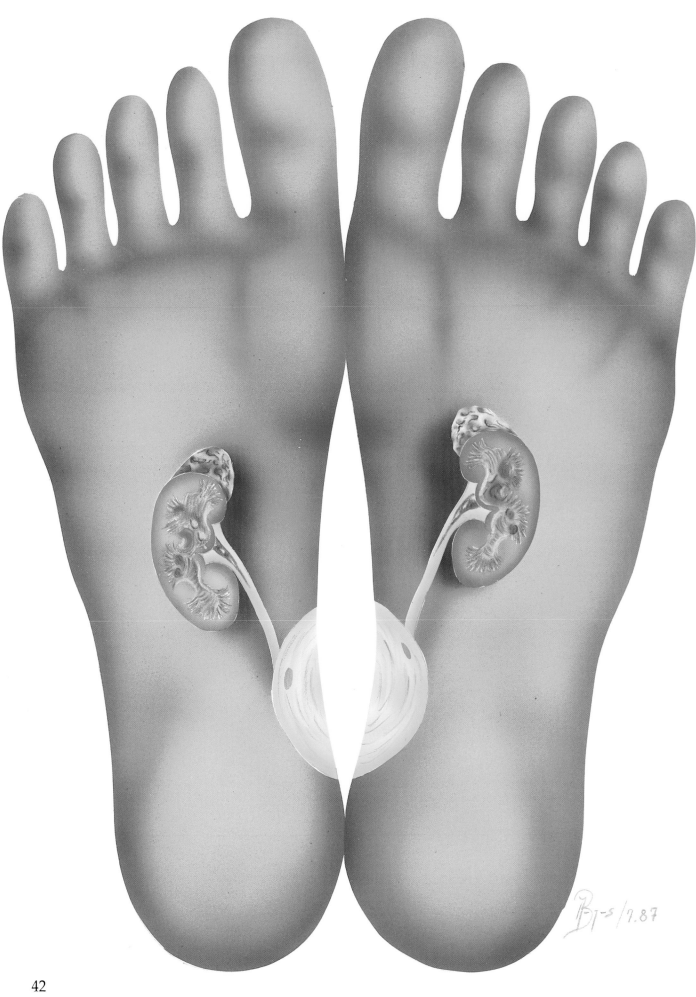

42

Foot Reflexology for Kidney and Bladder Disorders (Cross-Section View)

In my practice, I see many people who are suffering from pain, who are bent over and cramped up. They complain of extreme back pain (all the way to the pelvic region) that often extends into their legs.

After an intensive reflex-zone massage on the soles of their feet (the area of the kidneys and adrenal glands, ureter and bladder), a subsequent massage on the spinal column reflex zone (the area of the lumbar vertebrae and sacrum), and a light activation of the uterus and ovaries in the case of women and the prostate gland and testicles in the case of men, these patients are largely pain-free. In 80 percent of the cases the symptoms disappeared after a single massage session, even when they had persisted for a long time!

What had happened? The nerve pathways to the organ had been blocked, and there was an imbalance between supply and disposal. Massaging the reflex zones sent an impulse via the nervous system to the organs in question, which then relaxed. Afterward, the organs began to function normally again and the pain disappeared. No matter what the problem is in this area, it's necessary to massage at least three times a week—even when the body is free of pain—until the reflex-zone points are free of pain.

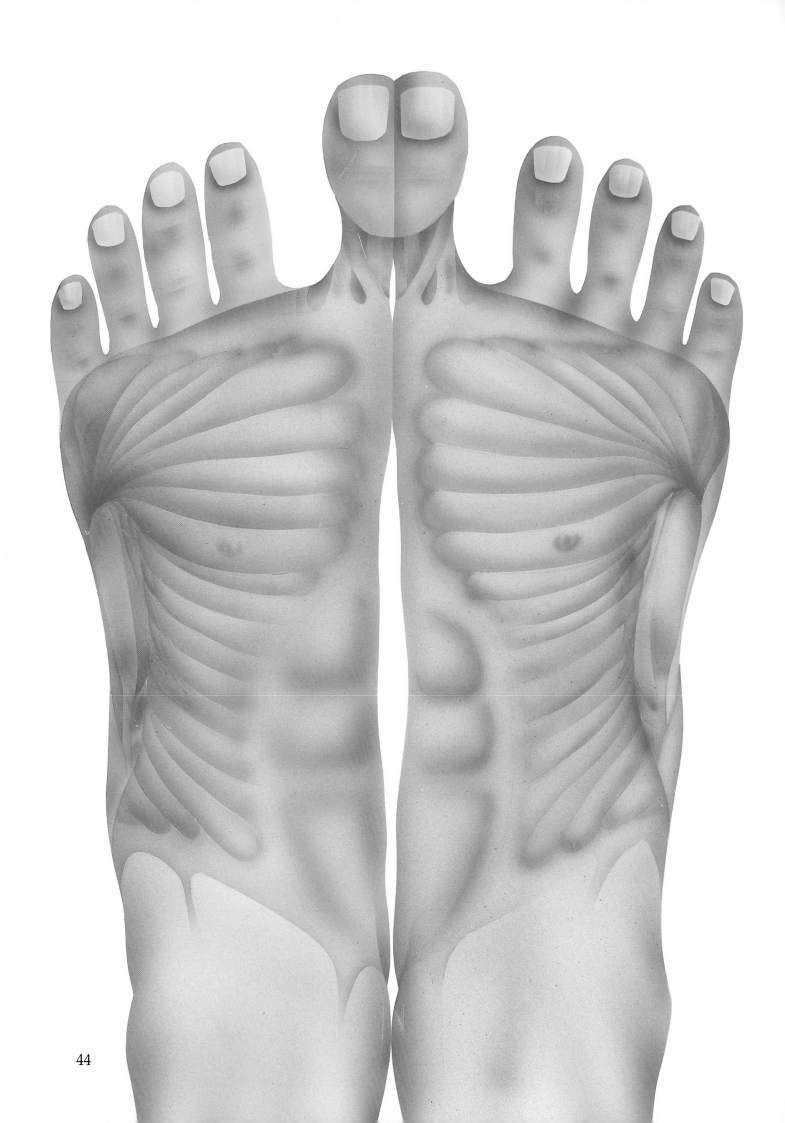

44

Foot Reflexology for the Muscles of the Front of the Body

At left you can see the frontal view of a man. For clarity, the big toes have been reversed. The head zone is distinctly visible: chin zone, neck muscles, larynx, shoulders, chest, upper arms, stomach muscles, loins, and groin.

When problems arise in these areas, the corresponding zones on the feet—or in emergencies on the hands—should be initially massaged for twenty minutes (ten minutes of massage, five-minute pause, ten minutes of massage). When the injuries are recent and there are no open wounds, one massage session will usually suffice. If there are open wounds, a doctor's care is advised.

For follow-up treatment, ten minutes of massage will do.

Important: Recent injuries are those no more than two days old. The more recent the injury, the more quickly it can be healed. The reflex zones of bruises and strains can be massaged at four- to five-hour intervals. For example, if a strain or bruise is massaged in the morning, afternoon, and evening, the patient is often back to normal the following day, even if the bruise is deep. It is important that you proceed with a lot of sensitivity. First, you should feel for hardness and knots in the reflex zones. It's crucial to locate the exact site of pain.

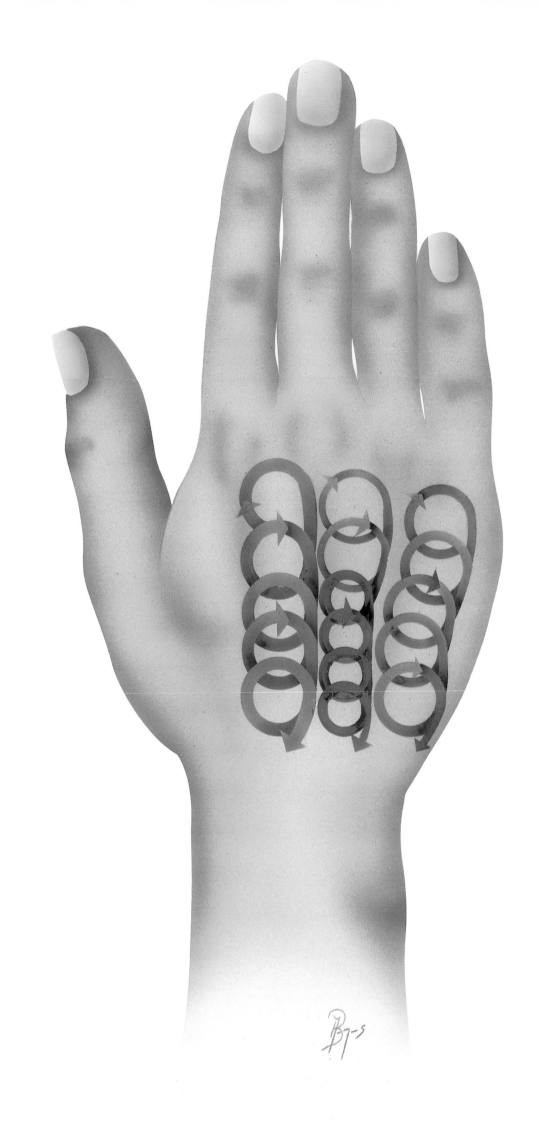

Massage Instructions for Slow-Healing Wounds

It sometimes happens that wounds refuse to close or are slow to heal. Reflex-zone massage has been used to speed the healing process, even in difficult cases. Aside from an intensive foot or hand massage—depending on where the wound is—there are also other massage possibilities that you might find useful.

• For foot injuries, try hand massage on the corresponding zones. The illustration at left shows one method of hand massage, stroking in a spiral motion from knuckle to wrist.
• For leg injuries, try arm massage in the corresponding area.
• For hand injuries, try foot massage in the corresponding zones.
• For arm injuries, try leg massage (or foot massage) in the corresponding area.
• For injuries in areas other than those mentioned above, try foot and hand massage in the corresponding zones.

However, all of this should be done only after you've consulted a doctor. Moreover, you should be treated by a trained, first-class masseur. The wounds will occasionally react with extreme pain or itchiness, in which case, your doctor should be notified.

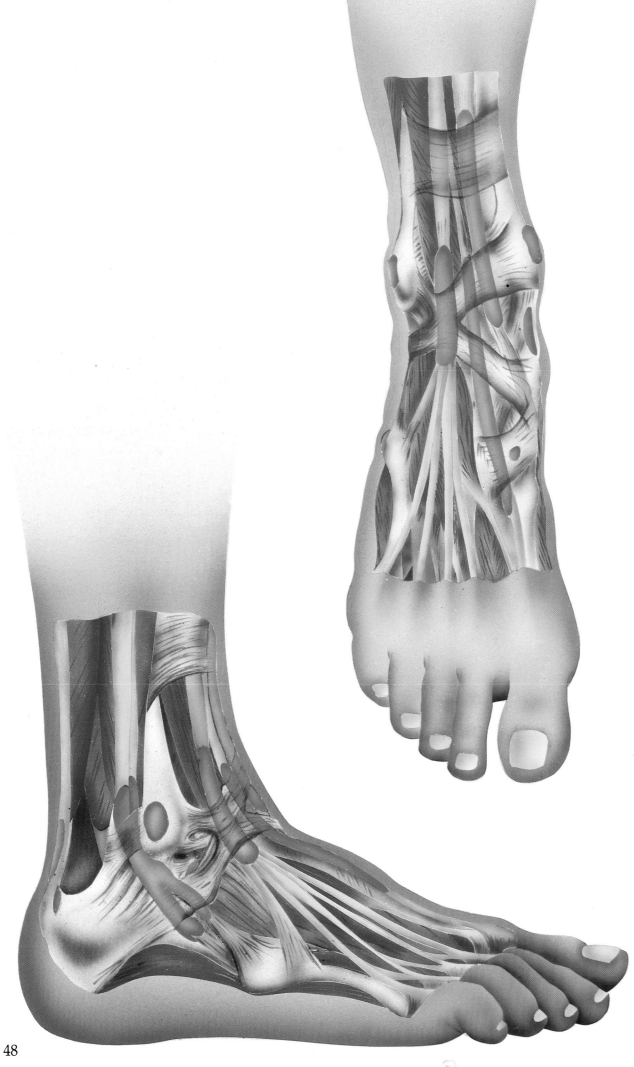

48

The Tendons of the Foot

When there is soreness in the lower legs, the lower arms should be massaged, and when there is soreness in the thighs, the upper arms should be massaged. Other massage options are suggested in the illustration shown below. Note the connection between the calf and the area behind the ball of the foot, and between the thigh and the area near the heel of the foot.

Recommendation: Men and women who work with typewriters, computers, cash registers, and the like should have their partners massage the tendons of the feet and lower legs daily as a precautionary measure against soreness in the tendons of the hands and arms. A massage of fifteen to twenty minutes should be sufficient to avoid problems; and can be employed as a first-aid measure if severe soreness develops in the hands and arms at work.

Note: Tendinitis can be avoided! Just think how many lost days of work you can eliminate.

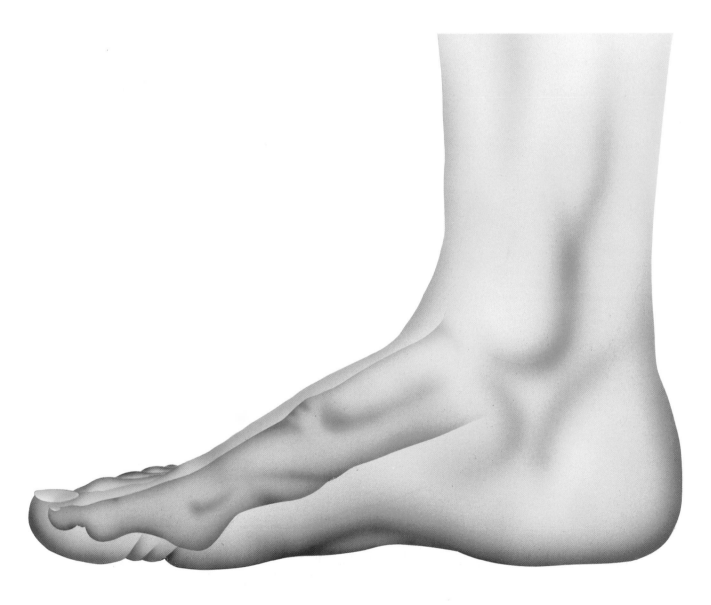

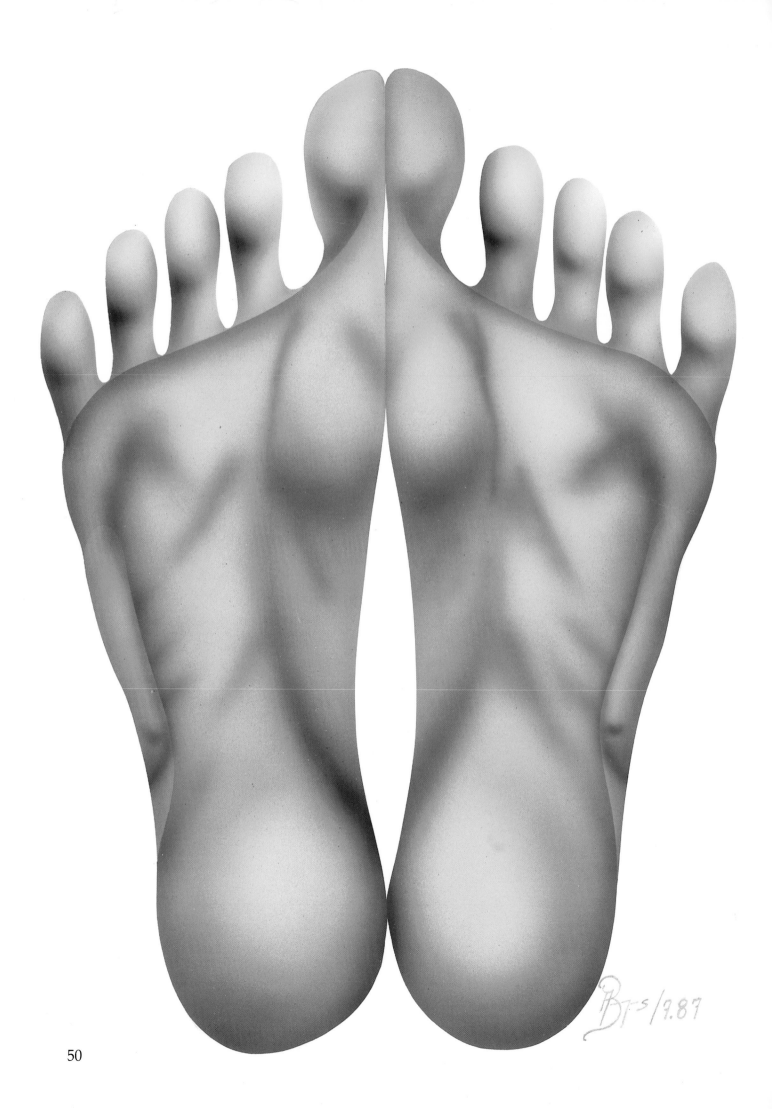

Foot Reflexology for Back Muscles

Here in the soles of the feet you see the rear view of a person sitting. If you look at the heels, you'll see the person's buttocks. On the outside of the feet are the upper arms. Further up you can make out the shoulders and finally the head, which is clearly recognizable in the reversed big toes.

If you look closely at the center portion of the illustration, you will see the back of the neck and the bulge of the lower cervical vertebrae. And if you look very closely, you'll be able to see another pair of buttocks just under the basal joint of the big toes. The arches of the feet show the backs of the thighs.

When you have soreness in the shoulder, back of the neck, or arms, the corresponding reflex zones of the foot should be vigorously massaged. It doesn't matter if it hurts—after several massage sessions the musculature will become limber.

Reactions: After foot massage, your muscles might ache, which is a good sign (indicating improved circulation). Don't forget to limber the basal joint of the big toe. In this illustration you can clearly see that the basal joint of the big toe is also the reflex zone for the lumbar vertebra and affects the buttocks and thighs.

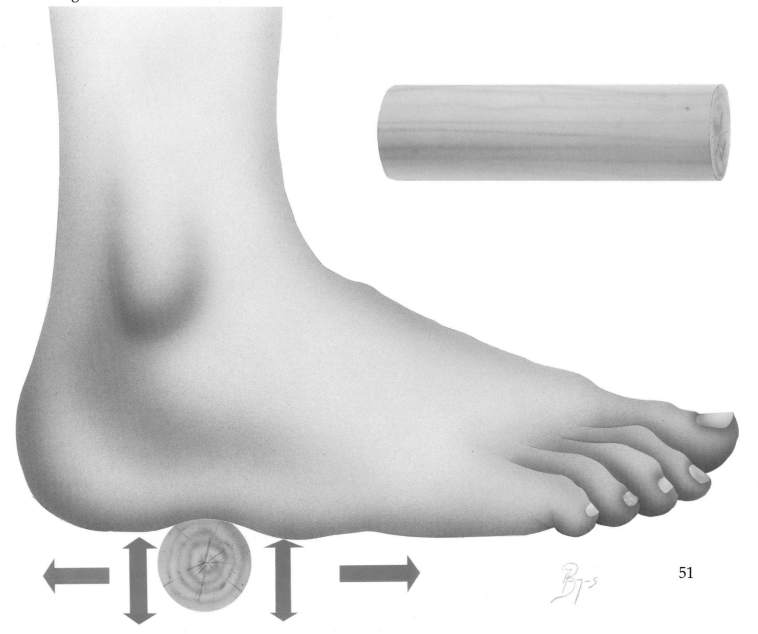

51

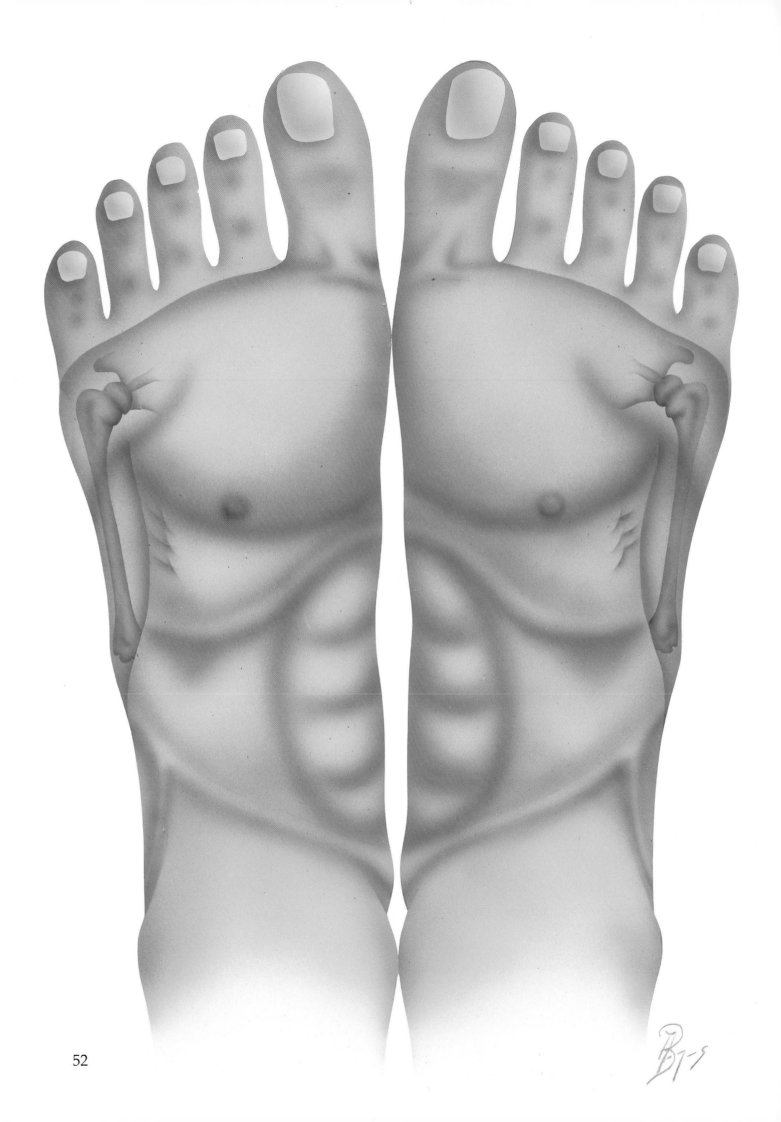

52

Foot Reflexology for the Muscles of the Front of the Body, and for Abdominal Surgery

After operations in the abdominal region (appendectomy, et cetera), the corresponding reflex zones—as shown in the illustrations of the foot—should be massaged in an effort to avoid or reduce scarring and tearing at the site of the incision, and to help the wounds to heal more quickly.

Following abdominal surgery, it is of the utmost significance that the joints and internal organs be reached via massage of the reflex zones. The illustration at left and those throughout the book will show you exactly where you have to massage. After suffering broken bones or torn ligaments, muscles, and tendons, use reflex-zone massage to reduce pain more quickly and speed the healing process. If you cannot do self-massage, or if you do not have a regular massage partner, now is the time to hire a good masseur. If need be, simply take this book with you when you go for treatment.

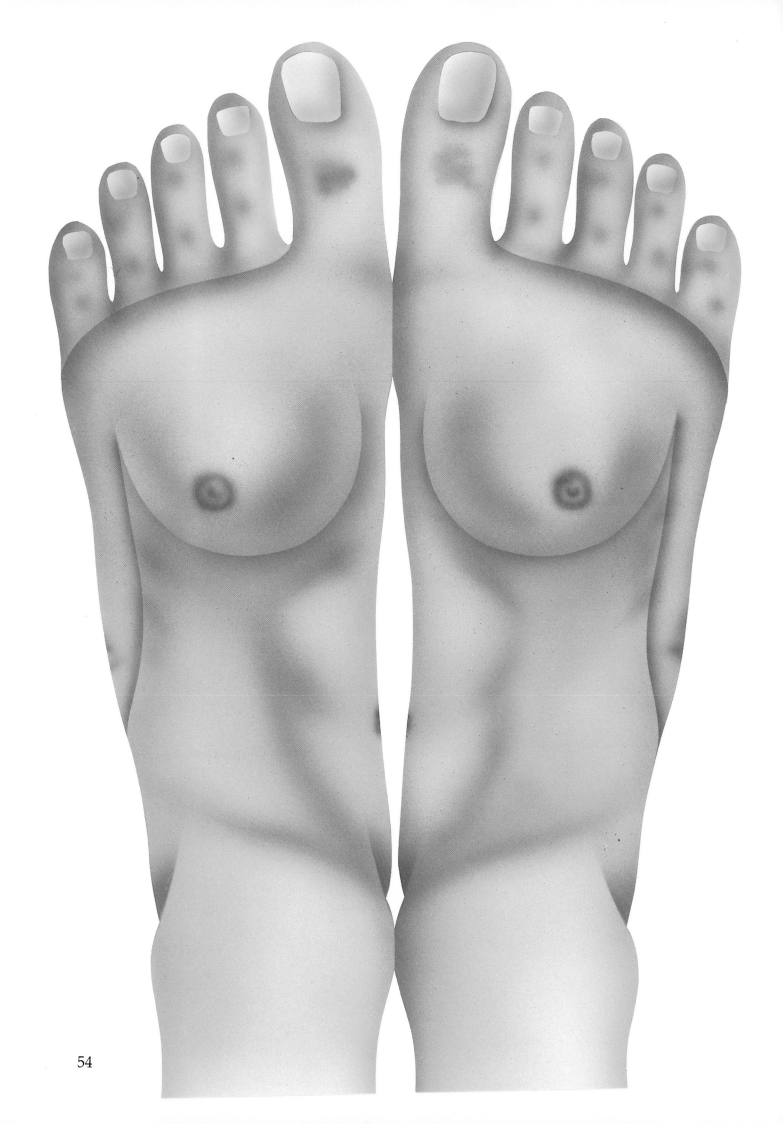

Foot Reflexology for the Breasts

We know through practical experience that bruises, strains, and hardness on parts of the body also cause hardness in the corresponding reflex zones. So it's only natural that any changes in a woman's breasts will be reflected in her hands and feet. The illustration at left and the one on page 56 show the foot reflex zones that correspond to the breasts. These areas can be massaged to "feel" for potential problems, or to help alleviate a current condition. I stress, however, that foot massage is not a substitute for regular checkups and examination by a physician.

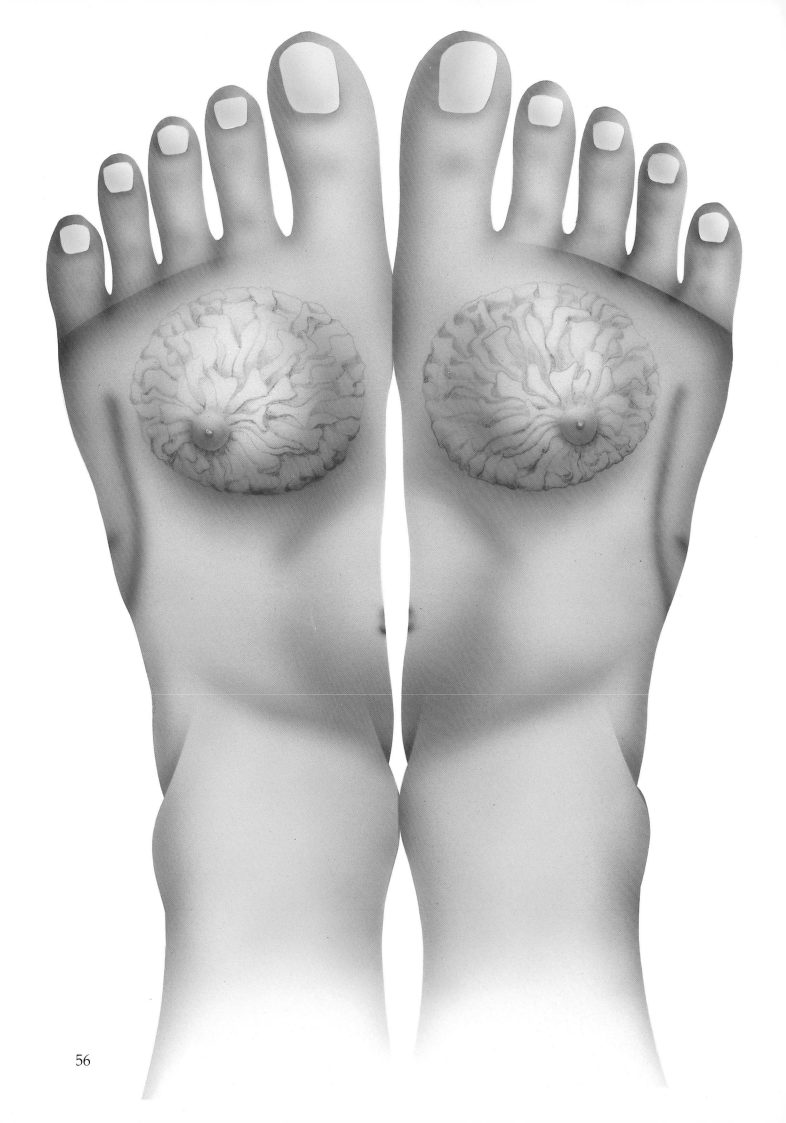

Foot Reflexology for the Mammary Glands

I'm always sad when I hear of women being operated on for problems in their breasts or lower abdomen. Through regular practice of reflex-zone massage, such problems might have been prevented.

It's important that no lumps form in the reflex zones for the breasts and mammary glands. However, if you do detect swelling, hardness, or even lumps, don't panic. If you notice a lump in the breast itself or in the reflex zones for the breast, you should be examined by a doctor immediately. Speak with him or her about reflex-zone massage, and then work with your massage partner or a good masseur and try to have the lump massaged away. Of course, you must also follow the instructions of your physician for treatment.

It has been my experience that if the masseur succeeds in massaging away the lump in the breast's reflex zones, the lump in the breast itself will also disappear. The same procedure is followed with disorders of the lymph nodes.

Important: *Always* consult a doctor, who has the last word! Also refer to the illustrations on pages 32, 34, and 58.

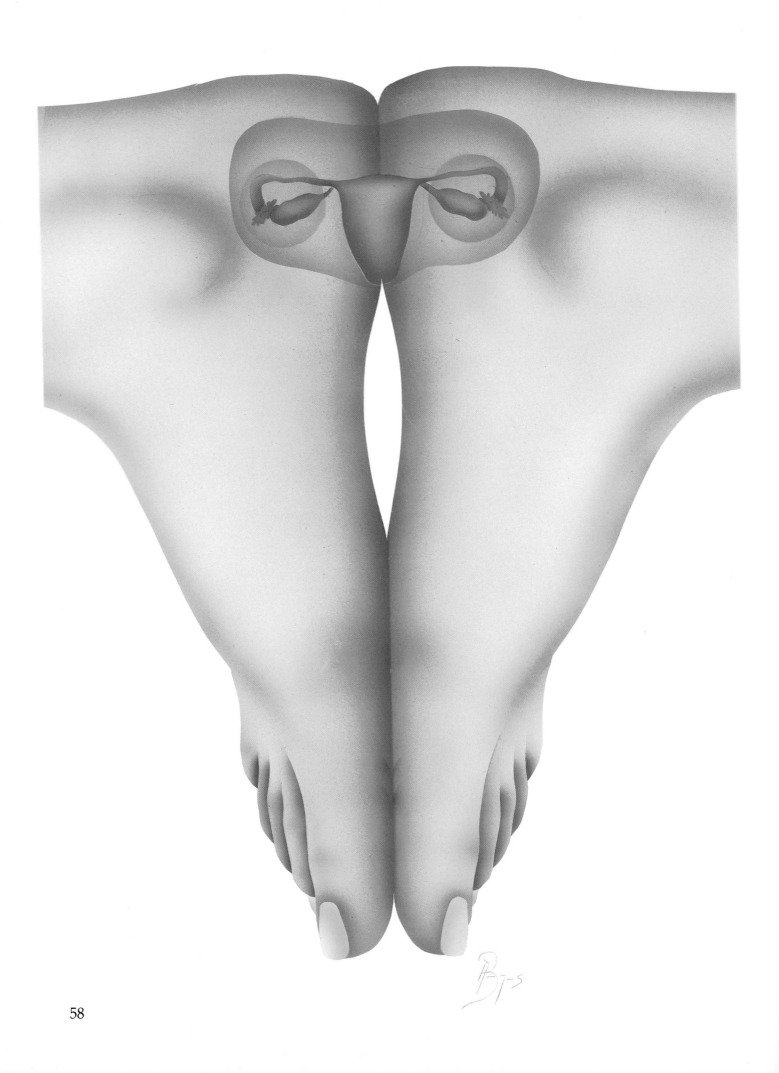

Foot Reflexology for the Uterus and Ovaries

The problems typical of females frequently begin in early childhood, but certainly no later than during the onset of puberty: pain, nausea, listlessness, irritability, and often even depression. In many cases, these problems are compounded by splitting headaches (migraines). To put it simply, there is a hormonal imbalance.

Massage: You should first try to limber the cervical vertebrae (basal joint of big toe).

Please refer to the illustration on page 14. If you have problems with your uterus or ovaries, massage the areas shown on the illustration at left. For disorders of the kidneys, ureter, and bladder massage the areas shown on pages 40 and 42. If all of the points are massaged using thumb pressure, a pleasantly warm sensation will spread throughout the body, and pain in the lower abdomen should generally disappear within a few minutes.

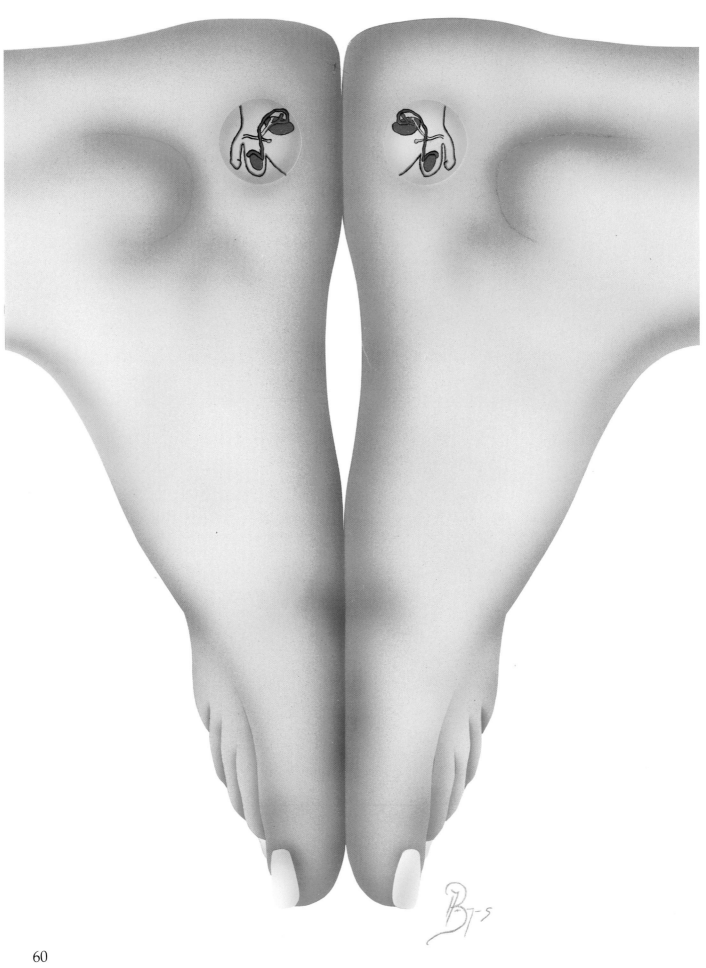

Foot Reflexology for the Prostate and Testicles

The same reflex zone applying to the uterus and ovaries in a woman corresponds to the prostate gland and testicles in a man. Just as this zone is critical to a woman, it is of the utmost importance to a man. Prophylactic massage of these points can help prevent prostate trouble and disorders of the testicles.

Even if you already have discomfort in these areas, the zones can be massaged successfully and surgery can possibly be avoided even in difficult cases.

Important: Reflex-zone massage is not a substitute for regular checkups and examination by a physician. If you have or suspect you have a problem in this area, see your doctor immediately. Speak to him or her about reflex-zone massage and then enlist the help of a massage partner or masseur.

When an operation simply can't be avoided, reflex-zone massage should be applied following surgery.

Treatment: Always massage the designated zone by pressing with your thumbs. It's important that the area of the kidneys and adrenal glands as well as the ureter and bladder are massaged as directed (see the illustrations on pages 40 and 42). The massage should last about three minutes per point; apply pressure massage using the thumbs.

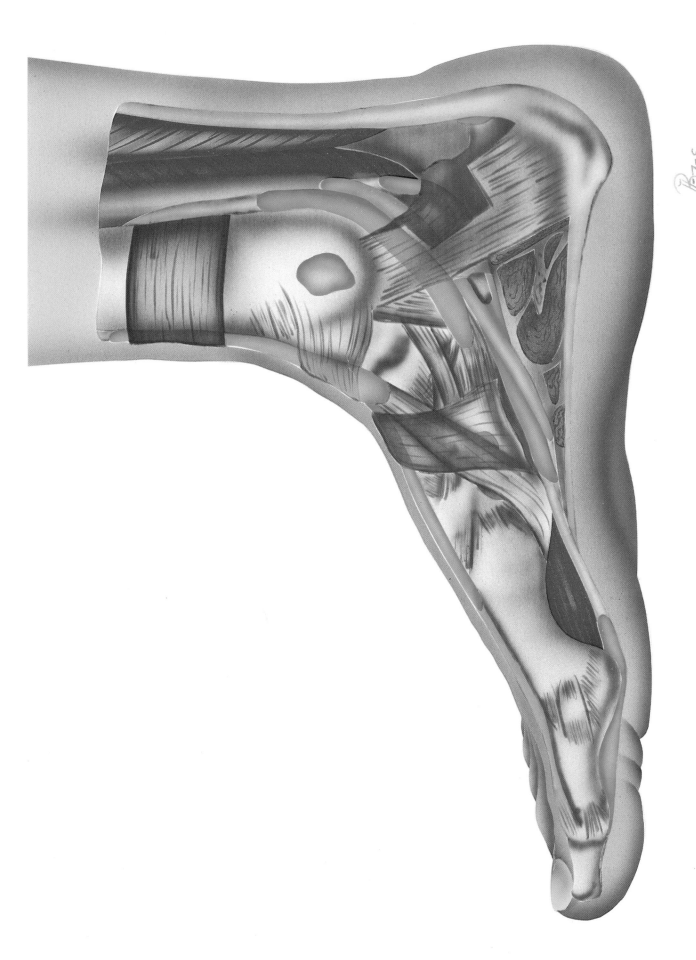

Is the Foot in the Foot or Is the Leg in the Foot?

Nonsense? Not at all! Just look at the illustrations carefully. The big toe, including the basal joint, definitely corresponds to the foot and Achilles tendon.

Connected to that is clearly a leg, and the ankle corresponds to the hip, the heel to the buttocks. When there is trouble with these zones, you can be sure the corresponding joints and body parts are affected!

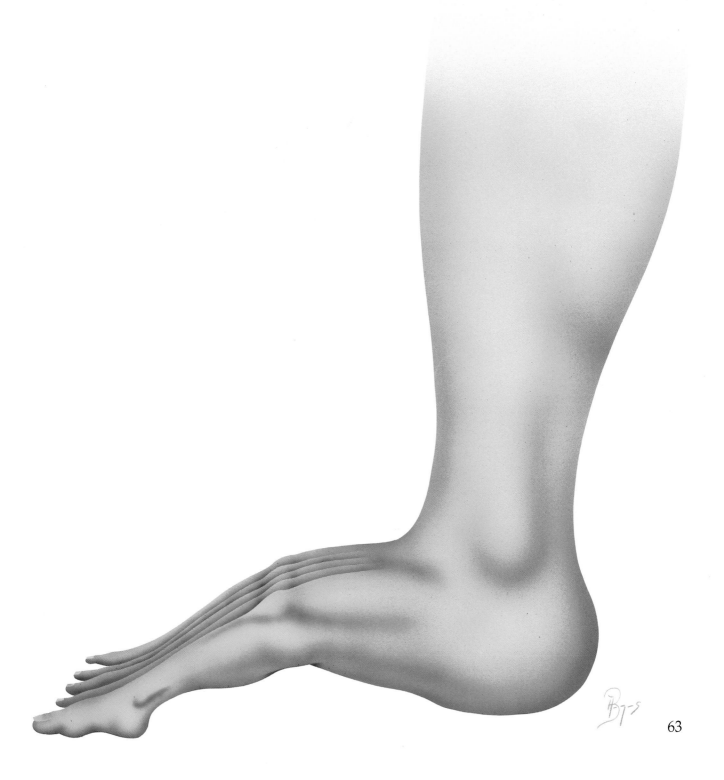

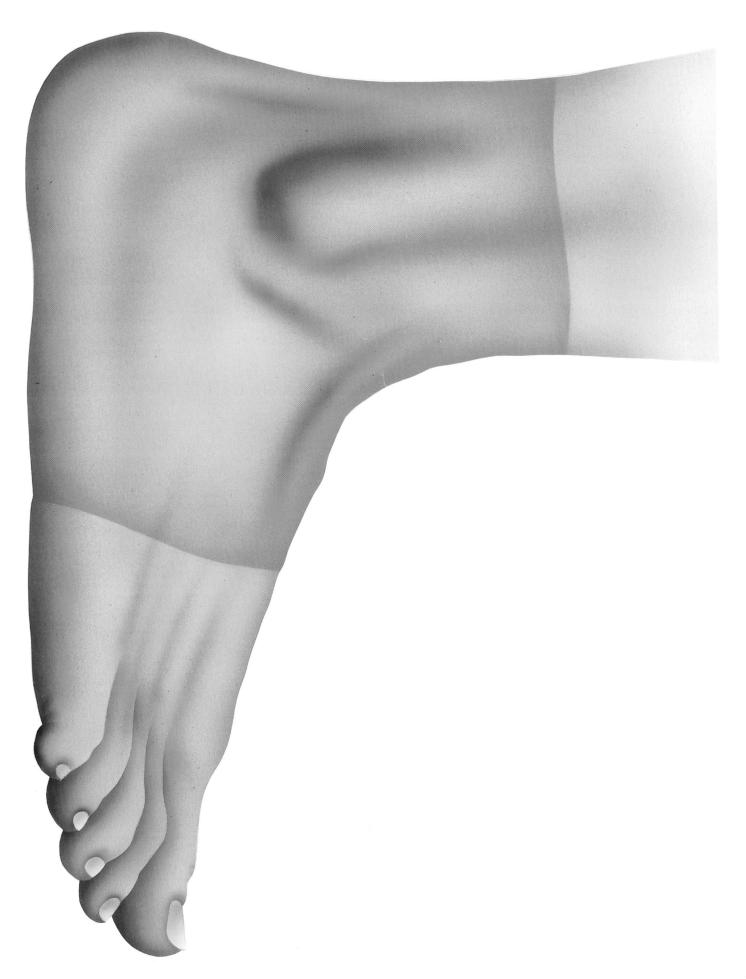

64

Reflexology for the Outside of the Knee

The knee, one of the most injury-prone joints, can be activated at several points using reflex-zone massage. The illustration at left indicates that the reflex zones for the outside of the knee are found in the heel, ankle, and metatarsus (the five bones between the ankle and toes). Other reflex zones for the outside of the knee are the elbow, the basal joints of the big toe and the thumb, and the rest of the toe and finger joints.

Whenever there's the slightest sign of knee trouble, it's advisable to massage the elbow—that is, the adjacent muscles of the upper and lower arm (feel for hardness). With light massage of the elbow, the knee will relax and become better supplied with blood.

When the knee problems are not so recent, the heel and entire foot—or, more precisely, both feet—should be massaged in addition to the elbow. The sensitive areas are the trouble spots and must therefore be massaged more vigorously.

The knee zones on the metatarsus are the reflex zones for the meniscus and the crucial ligaments. Careful massage will stimulate the blood circulation and make the knee more mobile.

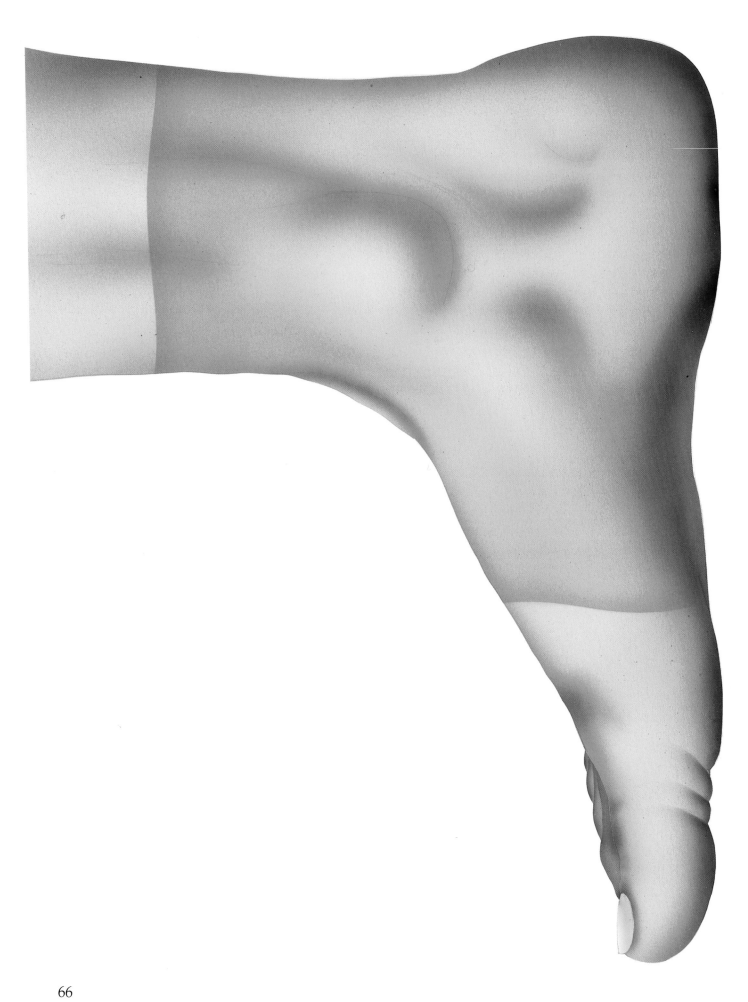

Reflexology for the Inside of the Knee

The illustration at left indicates that the reflex zones for the inside of the knee are found in the inside heel, ankle, and metatarsus (the five bones between the ankle and toes) area. Other reflex zones for the inside of the knee are the elbow, wrist, thenar (bulge at base of thumb), basal joints of fingers, and metacarpus (the five bones between wrist and fingers).

When you massage a reflex zone for the inner knee, don't be afraid if you suddenly feel acute pain in your knee or in the surrounding muscles. The increased circulation can cause pressure simply because some blood vessels aren't clear. When the disposal of waste products or possibly hardened hematomas begins, the nervous system reacts. And that's a good sign. The pain can last several days, particularly when the injuries are not recent, but then they should eventually vanish. If there is no improvement, however—which is not to be expected—you should see your doctor without delay.

Needless to say, you should always go to the doctor immediately when you've had an accident. If the doctor determines that nothing has been broken or torn, you can recover your physical fitness with reflex-zone massage. If you've had surgery, you can test reflex-zone massage as a post-operative treatment.

If you massage well and sufficiently—never the injured area, of course—you'll soon notice improvement. Your doctor can supervise the process.

Experience has shown that the post-operative application of reflex-zone massage achieves nearly optimal results. Scars are less likely to tear, and hematomas and other post-operative problems more quickly disappear (presuming surgery was successful). In short, the knee should become mobile, pain-free, and able to carry all your weight again.

A trained therapist is best equipped to practice reflex-zone massage, but for the layperson, practice makes perfect!

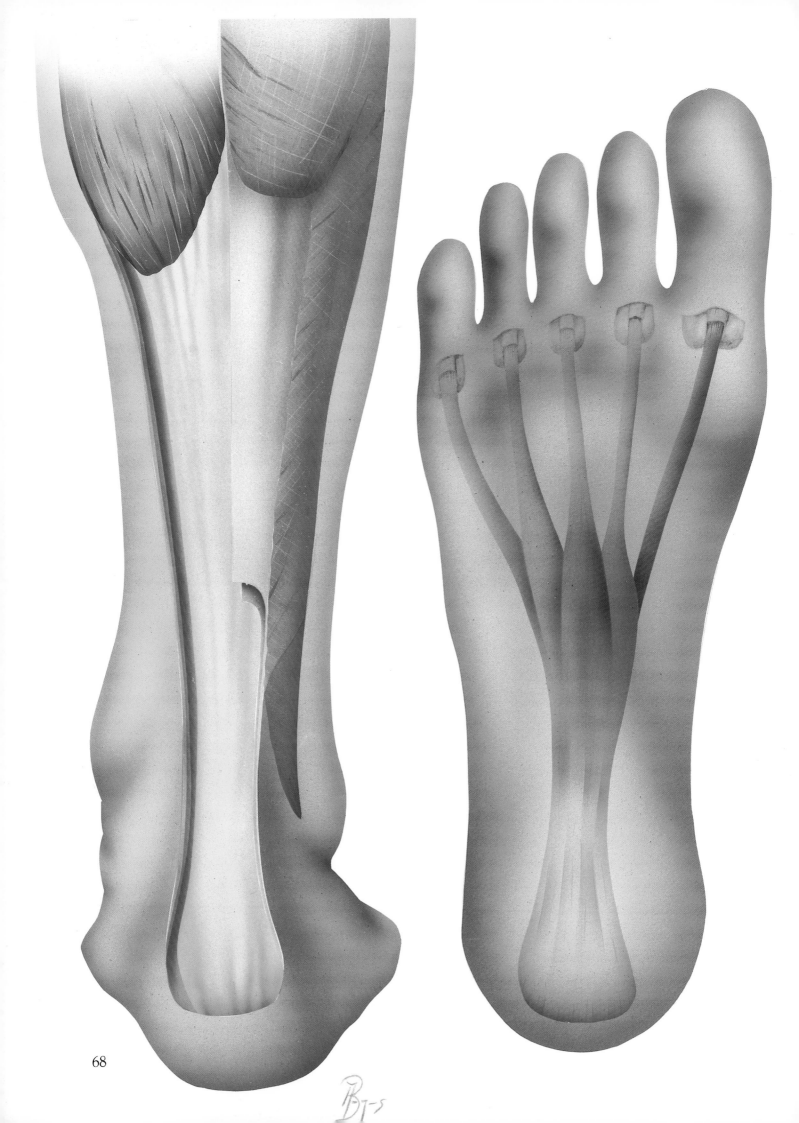

68

Foot Reflexology for the Achilles Tendon

When you have problems with an Achilles tendon—which are generally quite unpleasant and painful—massage the tendon tracts pictured on the sole of the foot.

If you look closely at the two illustrations at left, you'll see the correspondence between the tendons. The reflex zone for the outer Achilles tendon extends from the heel to the middle of the foot. The individual tendon tracts are the reflex zones for the inner part of the Achilles tendon.

Treatment: Never massage the injured areas. First massage the individual zones relatively softly. Massage more vigorously (depending on the pain threshold) only when the zones don't react so painfully. Always press all of the reflex zones for the Achilles tendons with your thumb.

You'll notice that some zones react quite strongly. They are precisely the main points that should be massaged more intensively until the pain subsides. The Achilles tendon will warm up, which is an unmistakable sign of improved blood circulation. The pain will be eased.

You can massage as directed following surgery on the Achilles tendon or after a tear or an accident. You and your doctor will likely be amazed at how soon you'll be able to stand normally and walk without pain again.

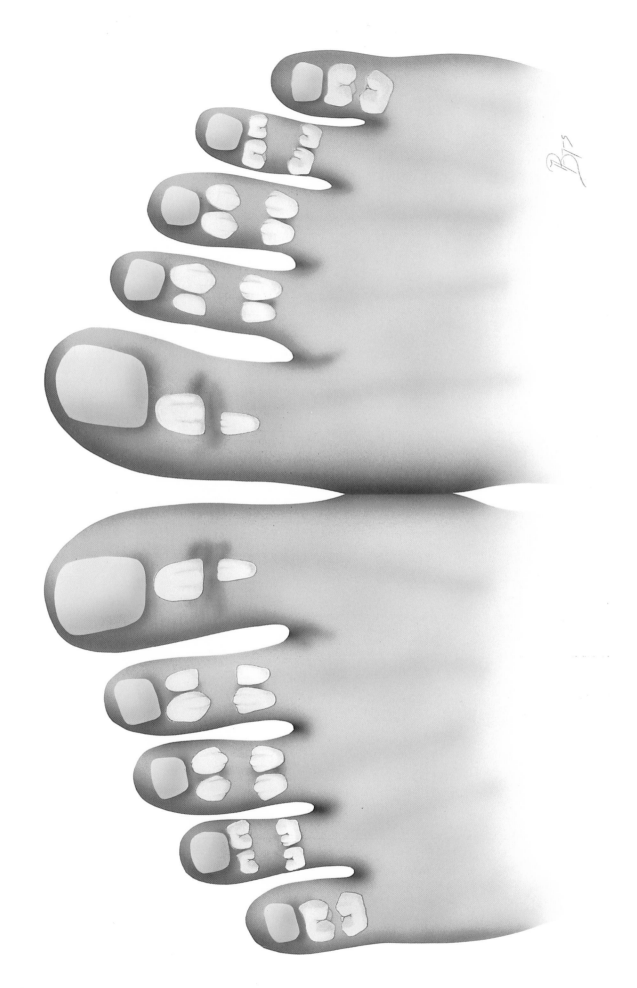

Foot Reflexology for the Teeth

Reflex-zone massage can be quite helpful here in taking care of the teeth and gums. In the illustration at left, you can see the teeth pictured on the top sides of the toes. When you massage these areas, you automatically massage the upper and lower jaws as well. Toothaches or pain in the gums and jaws can often be relieved in this way. When you have a toothache, locate the culprit and press (pump) the corresponding spot on the toe with your thumb. It will hurt terribly, but in most cases the pain will subside. **This method is meant only as first aid and not as a substitute for seeing a dentist!** If you massage as a precautionary measure, the teeth and gums will be well supplied with blood and you'll avoid tooth and gum and jaw diseases.

Should pea-sized red spots appear on the top sides of the toes, you can assume there is a problem with the corresponding teeth or gum or jaw zone. Go to the dentist immediately for an examination.

If you always keep your toes soft and supple, you shouldn't have to worry much about your teeth.

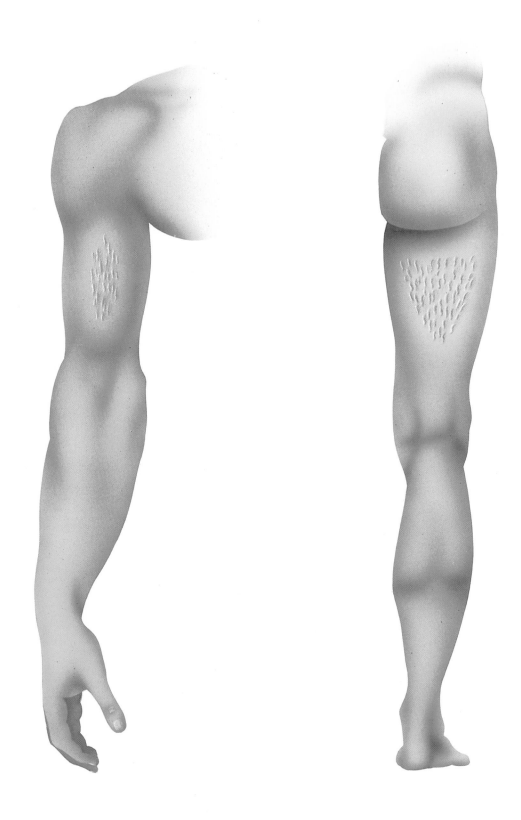

Reflexology for Strains and Ruptured Muscles

Strains, ruptured muscles, and hematomas can usually be cured immediately if they are recent. Any injury not yet forty-eight hours old is a recent one.

As shown in the illustrations at left, the thigh corresponds to the upper arm and vice versa.

The massage should be performed with care. The muscle must be well raised (see the illustration on page 75). The knots can be felt and lightly moved using the thumb and index finger. This should always be done by applying pressure upward (toward the shoulder when massaging the arm, and toward the buttocks when massaging the leg).

Massage lightly for ten minutes, take a five-minute break, then massage vigorously for ten minutes.

If hardness remains, the injury was either old or the muscle was tight before the injury. In that case, the massage must be repeated, but the follow-up treatments should not exceed ten minutes (don't overstimulate the area). The massage is painful so the patient must indicate when he's reached his limit. Everyone has a different threshold of pain.

I've achieved my greatest success with this sort of massage—in all branches of sports and industry, in amateur and professional sports leagues. When the athletes were massaged in time (in cases of recent injuries), they returned to the game immediately afterward and often led their teams on to victory.

One thing is always important: The injury must no longer hurt after the massage. If the athlete feels no pain, he can safely resume playing.

When an athlete has been seriously injured but cannot afford to be sidelined for long, he may be massaged every five to six hours—but no longer than ten minutes during the follow-up sessions.

Never overstimulate a reflex zone! Otherwise, it can no longer be massaged. By following this rule you can promote quick healing of hemotomas, tightness, strains, and ruptured muscles.

Reactions: The injured area will warm up and may even become painful and twinge. That's a good sign, however, because it indicates that blood circulation is optimal.

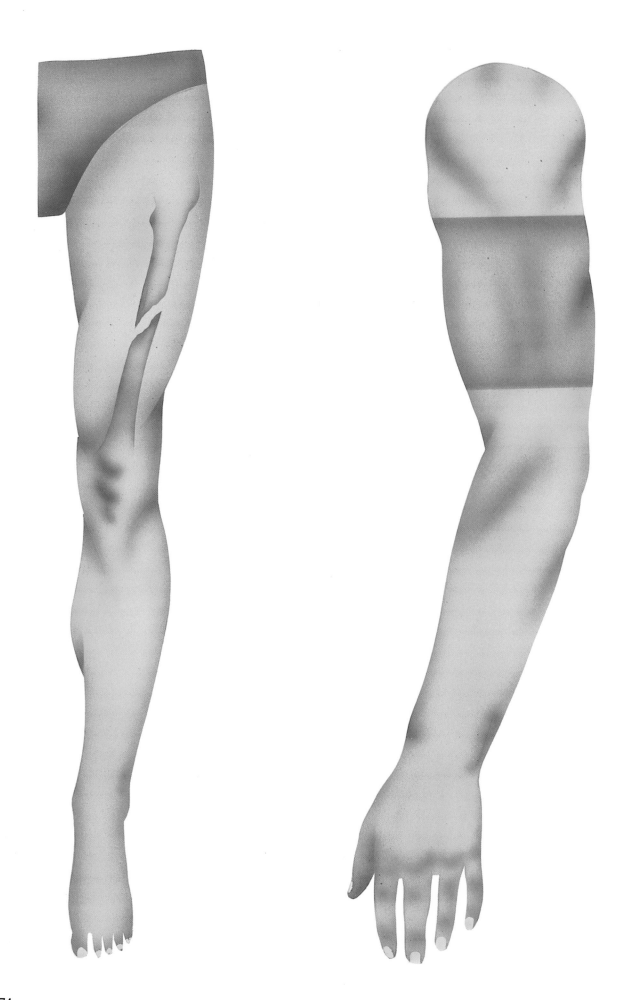

Reflexology for Broken Bones

The point where the leg was broken is the point where the arm should be massaged, and vice versa.

Treatment: First find the problem zone and lightly massage it for about ten minutes. Take a five-minute break and then massage for another ten minutes, this time with a little more pressure. You should repeat this procedure daily until the problems have disappeared. The illustration below shows the proper massage grip.

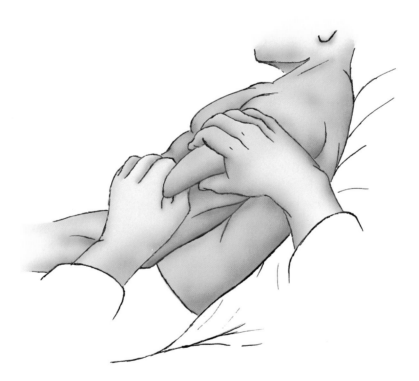

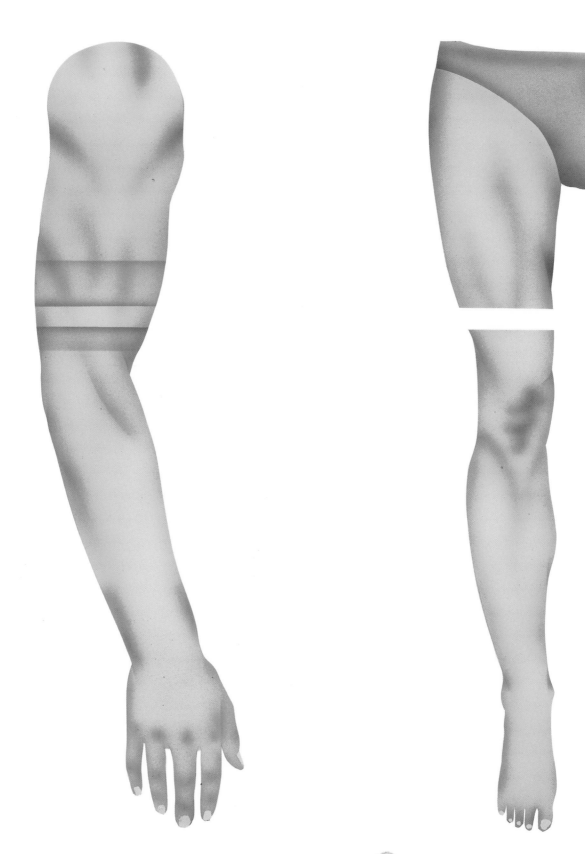

Reflex-Zone Massage for Amputations

Unfortunately, amputations are not uncommon. And problems of the most varied sort often arise after the operation. I've found that massaging the corresponding reflex zone (in the arm for a leg amputation; in the leg for an arm amputation) brings rapid relief after surgery. The wounds heal more quickly, there is little scarring and no inflammation, and you are spared phantom pain.

It is essential that the diseased area itself not be touched! The initial massage session should last about twenty minutes, the following sessions ten minutes. Reflex-zone massage may also bring relief of pain from old surgical scars and war injuries. The irritation and swelling and pain caused by wearing a prosthesis may also disappear through reflex-zone massage.

Important: Massage softly at first, then with more pressure. Simply feel for the swelling in the reflex zones and massage it away. In cases of old amputations and injuries, you may find hardness in the reflex zones that can slowly be massaged away. The first massage session should be about twenty minutes; later sessions should be ten minutes in duration.

Note: Beware of shrapnel! If there is any, always consult your doctor first.

Amputations

The point where the arm was severed is the point where the leg should be massaged, and vice versa. **Important:** A painful stump, phantom pain, pain caused by artificial limbs, or just general pain from wounds can be eliminated by massaging the corresponding reflex zones.

Post-operative massage of the reflex zones accelerates healing and prevents inflammation, the hardening of scars, and general discomfort. The first treatment for amputation should consist of a ten-minute massage followed by a five-minute break, followed by a ten-minute massage.

Old scars and hardened areas may react painfully during or after the massage. Such reactions will quickly cease, however, if the massage is practiced regularly. The hardness will disappear and the scars will soften simply because the zones are well supplied with blood.

Note: When there is a blood clot in the leg, the leg *must not* be massaged directly. In that case, treatment proceeds via the reflex zone on the arm.

Follow-up massages should be of ten-minute duration. You can massage daily, and you should massage at least three times a week until the problems disappear. Then massage once a week as a precautionary measure.

Reflexology for Babies and Small Children

Babies frequently have perplexing problems. They often vomit, cry, sleep poorly or not at all, and have cramps. No medicine helps, nor does tea or anything else. In short, both the baby and the parents are distressed, especially since the little one isn't able to say what's wrong.

The time-honored approach of letting the baby cry itself to sleep is dangerous and can lead to real illness.

Do you still remember the birth of your baby? When a newborn first sees the light of day, it's given a spank so that it cries and begins to breathe deeply. And everyone is happy to hear a strong little voice. Then the baby is carefully washed, weighed, and wrapped.

Now take a look at the wild. How do animal mothers treat their new offspring? After giving birth, the mother carefully licks her young, giving them a thorough rubdown. The mother's tongue massages the little bodies, normal functioning begins, hunger sets in, and the mother can start nursing.

Certainly there are many differences between humans and animals, but we can learn quite a bit from their behavior. To make my point, could foot reflexology promote more normal, harmonious functioning in our babies and children? My experience says yes, it can.

Since it's unable to walk, a newborn needs to be activated. If you massage your baby's feet for just a minute each day, you provide important beneficial stimulation. In my practice I have observed that babies given regular foot massage have very few problems, cry only when they are hungry, grow splendidly, and sleep soundly.

It goes without saying, of course, that you should have your baby looked at by a doctor—regular checkups are a must. But you can employ reflex-zone massage without worry as a kind of first aid.

If your baby has cramps, for example, massage the soles of both of its feet in accordance with the illustrations for digestive tract on page 38. Your baby should calm down immediately (if it doesn't, consult your regular pediatrician).

Many babies get too much mucus in their bronchial tubes. A daily massage for one to two minutes per foot (see the illustration on the bronchial tubes, page 36) is helpful.

Tip: The feet of babies and small children normally feel very firm. Massage them vigorously, but don't squeeze them and, whatever you do, don't pull on their toes!

All of the illustrations in this book are equally applicable to babies and small children. Duration of massage: just one to two minutes per foot. You'll get very rapid results.

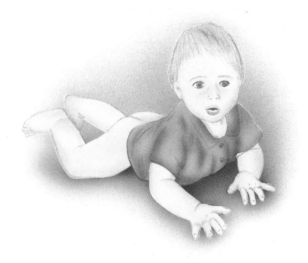

About the Author

Jürgen Jora was born in 1938 in Hamburg, Germany. He has made a name for himself as a sports masseur both in Germany and abroad with his spectacular successes using naturopathic treatments. His unique method of reflex-zone massage has both helped and healed numerous people, including many well-known top athletes. These successes are acknowledged by authorities in the field of classical medicine, who have been working together with Jürgen Jora for a long time. His method can be applied to practically all disorders and diseases of the human body.

Jürgen Jora's successes in healing have been frequently and enthusiastically reported in the newspaper, on radio, and on television. Now he's decided to speak for himself, presenting his decades of experience in an easy-to-grasp format and plain language to both laypersons and therapists. As Jürgen Jora writes, "One of mankind's most cherished dreams will come true for you: With just a few easy strokes, you'll be able to rid yourself of pain and the causes of disease!"

The large, colorful illustrations found in this book are the first of their kind and make the book especially valuable. Based on human anatomy, they make the body's reflex zones immediately clear even to the layperson and, together with the accompanying texts, are a proven means to regain and maintain health.

Because all the people seeking help cannot be treated in his practice in Hamburg, Germany, Jürgen Jora hopes this book will help to spread his method of reflex-zone massage.

Going Feet First

Reflexology is a massage science that benefits the whole body.

Humans have been stroking sore feet since the time of sandals and staffs, but a foot rub can be much more than just a mode of blissful relaxation. According to the holistic discipline of reflexology, your feet reflect the condition of your entire body, with specific spots linked to other body parts. Working these areas with thumbs or fingers can gently encourage the body to cure and strengthen itself, healing not just the prevailing symptoms but the person as a whole.

It doesn't seem logical that foot massage would provide overall therapeutic benefits, yet the concept that there are reflexes on the soles of the feet, the palms of the hands, and even the ears which correspond to organs and glands is not new; pictographs dating back to 2300 BC depict foot work being performed on satisfied recipients.

What is new is the widespread use and growing body of research on reflexology today: In Denmark, more than 3,500 reflexologists work in medical settings, including hospitals, and large corporations commonly employ them for employees' benefit. In China, a recent study conducted at Beijing Medical University examined how type 2 diabetes could be treated with foot reflexology.

Though American doctors William Fitzgerald and Joe Shelby Riley, along with "The Mother of Reflexology," physiotherapist Eunice D. Ingham, developed the modern incarnation of reflexology back in the 1920s, the healing art is now enjoying a surge of recognition in the US. "Reflexology is

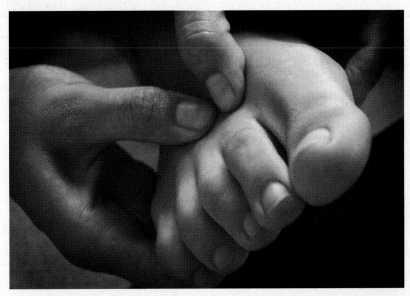

becoming more accepted as more people look to alternatives to allopathic [conventional] medicine," says Michael Rainone, president of the New York State Reflexologist Association (www.newyorkstate reflexology.org). "When first-timers try reflexology they cannot believe how good they feel."

Reflexology eases the symptoms of everyday ills and can effectively treat complaints as diverse as migraines, back pain, sleep disorders, PMS, hormonal imbalances, hypertension, circulatory issues and digestive disorders. "Basically, a disease is a blockage of energy in the body," says Rodney Mayfield, a certified reflexologist in Lancaster, New York. "Using reflexology, you can release blockages anywhere in the entire body."

Mayfield has witnessed dramatic improvement among his patients, including increased range of motion in stroke victims, lowered blood

pressure and remarkable changes in patients suffering from constipation. "I've had patients tell me that, after years of strenuous problems, they are easily eliminating every day," says Mayfield.

It is important for reflexology patients to provide a complete medical history prior to their first session. "You need to ask questions because people overlook or forget key issues," says Evelyn Bergdoll, LMT, a second-generation reflexologist with a practice in Burnham, Maine. "Generally, those issues are conditions that can be helped with reflexology."

Bergdoll has witnessed significant success with a variety of disorders, including conditions like back pain, that are often induced by stress. "Reflexology increases circulation and the flow of lymphatic fluid," she notes.

Bergdoll even found that reflexology helped her quit smoking, after attempting to quit cigarettes six

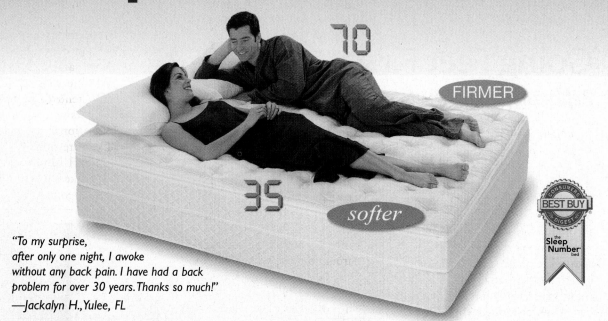
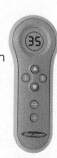

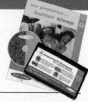

times on her own. "After just two weeks of reflexology treatments from my mother, I was able to stop smoking. The treatments purged my body of nicotine and toxins, and eliminated my cravings."

Playing Footsie

The science behind reflexology is based on "energy zones": Imagine your body is a giant gingerbread man divided lengthwise into 10 pieces. Every organ, muscle, bone, tendon, cell and ligament belongs to one of these zones, which all lead to the soles of your feet. Many also lead to reflex points in your hands and ears, but the feet are more receptive as they are not as compact. They also tend to accumulate more toxins as a result of gravity, which can be released from the body through the process. Plus, frankly, it just feels great to have your feet rubbed.

While a simple foot massage reduces stress and tension and encourages the body to strengthen itself, it does not provide the full, complex benefits of reflexology. Through the assistance of a certified reflexologist, or a guide map to the proper points, anyone can pick up the basics pretty quickly.

The most common technique is known as the "thumb walk." Bend your thumb at an approximately 45 degree angle and make tiny "steps" over a specific area (press, release, slide, repeat). Use the side of your thumb to apply steady, gentle pressure. You can also use the edge of your thumb and index fingers to take small "bites." This method allows you to direct pressure on a single point, since pressure is the key to effective reflexology. Sometimes, a point will be tender; it's important to work through the "hurt" over time, but if the area feels bruised or very painful, you are pressing too hard.

You can experiment with reflexology and build overall health simply by working your hands or feet for five to 15 minutes daily. You can also practice reflexology principles on common ailments. For instance, bouts of constipation can strike during times of stress or dietary change. Kneading your feet, breathing deeply and visualizing your intestines "relaxing" can act as an all-natural laxative. Get comfortable and work some lotion into your feet for five to 10 minutes, stroking and squeezing along the way. When your feet are feeling happy, locate the center of each sole, along the foot's arch. Press both thumbs in deeply, one at a time, and hold for three minutes.

At-home reflexology treatments can help relieve headaches and sinus conditions. The toes and fingers represent the head and neck on both the hands and feet. Use your thumb to "walk" over the surfaces of all toes, including the bottoms, tops and sides. Repeat two times on both feet until you feel some relief.

To learn more about reflexology, Bergdoll recommends *Feet First: A Guide to Foot Reflexology* (Fireside), featuring detailed charts, while Mayfield suggests *The Complete Illustrated Guide to Reflexology* (Element Books Ltd).

"You can find a wide variety of books to learn some simple techniques for working on your own feet," says Rainone. "Of course, there is no substitute for another human being touching your feet. Don't you agree?"

—Susan Weiner

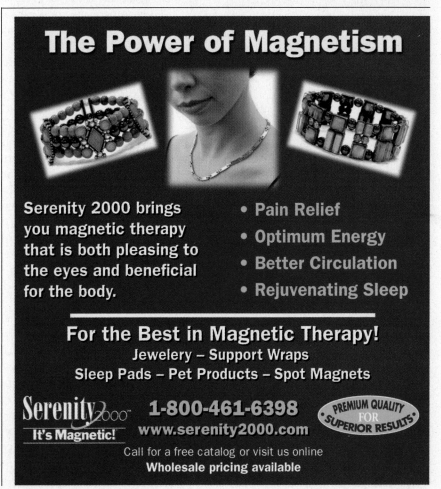

Sticking with Cinnamon

Exotic yet comforting, this spice adds delightful bite to any meal.

Hot apple cider and cinnamon is a classic combo for this time of year as leaves and temperatures fall together. And cinnamon is a classic kitchen staple, one that appears in nearly every pantry across the country.

But this old-school spice is the subject of new speculation: Research has found that cinnamon makes insulin more effective and

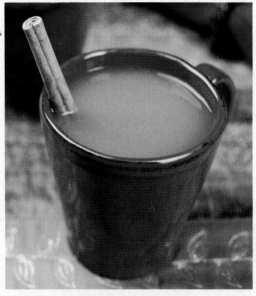

helps control blood sugar—which is good news for people with diabetes—and it may kill foodborne microbes. Sniffing cinnamon oil might even help ease road rage by reducing driver frustration!

Cinnamon's ability to beat up on bacteria—along with its exceptionally pungent scent and taste—may explain why it was treasured by the cream of European society in the Middle Ages, who used it to make spoiled meat go down more easily.

Eventually, a rising middle class meant rising demand for all spices, which led merchants across the seas to Ceylon (now known as Sri Lanka), where they found cinnamon's source: the bark of an evergreen tree, *Cinnamomum zeylanicum*. (In fact, most of what we call "cinnamon" in this country is actually cassia, a different species—*C. loureirii*—of the same tree.) Today, cinnamon and cassia are still harvested the traditional way, by peeling strips of bark that curl as they dry into sticks.

Most Americans know cinnamon as a welcome addition to baked goods and sweets (in Mexico, it's added to chocolate), and it certainly helps bring out fruit's natural sweetness, as in the recipe shown here. But cultures the world over have put the cassia tree's treasure to work in marinades and dressings for all sorts of meats, including poultry and fish. In addition, cinnamon imparts a delightful taste to beverages other than hot cider (it actually appears in many liqueurs).

When cooking with cinnamon, remember that the ground variety releases flavor more quickly than the whole spice, so use ground cinnamon in recipes that call for short cooking times or add it at the end of longer cooking times. Otherwise, stick with cinnamon sticks.

Like all spices, cinnamon starts losing its pep after being ground. Keep it in a dry, dark place and check frequently for loss of color or odor. To avoid introducing moisture into the bottle, don't shake cinnamon directly over a steaming pot. A smart alternative is to buy stick

cinnamon and grind it yourself in a spice mill.

Sometimes you just have to fall back on the tried-and-true. If you want to make both your taste buds and your insulin happy, turn to cinnamon's warm embrace.

—Lisa James

ET Recipe

Lucia's Poached Pears with Cinnamon and Prunes

- 3 slightly underripe Anjou pears
- 10 prunes
- 1 stick cinnamon
- 3 cloves
- 1 vanilla bean
- 2 strips lemon peel (organic preferred)
- 1 1/4 cups water
  ground cinnamon for garnish

1. Peel pears, place in heavy pot. Add other ingredients except for ground cinnamon.
2. Cover tightly and bring to a boil. Reduce heat to low and cook for 20 minutes, or until tender (test by piercing center of pears with a knife; if it passes easily, they're cooked).
3. Spoon into serving bowls and sprinkle with ground cinnamon. Serve warm or chilled.

Serves 3. Analysis per serving: 165 calories, 1.4g protein, 0.8g fat, 42g carbohydrates

Recipe courtesy of Spices of Life *by Nina Simonds (Knopf).*